Cambridge Elements ≡

Elements in Molecular Oncology
edited by
Edward P. Gelmann
University of Arizona

TARGETING ONCOGENIC DRIVER MUTATIONS IN LUNG CANCER

Matthew Lee
Montefiore Medical Center and Albert Einstein College of Medicine

Fawzi Abu Rous
Henry Ford Health System

Alain Borczuk
Weill Cornell Medicine

Stephen Liu
Lombardi Comprehensive Cancer Center, Georgetown University

Shirish Gadgeel
Henry Ford Health System

Balazs Halmos
Montefiore Medical Center and Albert Einstein College of Medicine

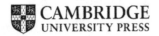

CAMBRIDGE
UNIVERSITY PRESS

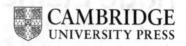

CAMBRIDGE
UNIVERSITY PRESS

Shaftesbury Road, Cambridge CB2 8EA, United Kingdom

One Liberty Plaza, 20th Floor, New York, NY 10006, USA

477 Williamstown Road, Port Melbourne, VIC 3207, Australia

314–321, 3rd Floor, Plot 3, Splendor Forum, Jasola District Centre,
New Delhi – 110025, India

103 Penang Road, #05–06/07, Visioncrest Commercial, Singapore 238467

Cambridge University Press is part of Cambridge University Press & Assessment,
a department of the University of Cambridge.

We share the University's mission to contribute to society through the pursuit of
education, learning and research at the highest international levels of excellence.

www.cambridge.org
Information on this title: www.cambridge.org/9781009336130

DOI: 10.1017/9781009336123

First published 2023

A catalogue record for this publication is available from the British Library.

ISBN 978-1-009-33613-0 Paperback
ISSN 2634-7490 (online)
ISSN 2634-7482 (print)

Targeting Oncogenic Driver Mutations in Lung Cancer

Elements in Molecular Oncology

DOI: 10.1017/9781009336123
First published online: January 2023

Matthew Lee
Montefiore Medical Center and Albert Einstein College of Medicine

Fawzi Abu Rous
Henry Ford Health System

Alain Borczuk
Weill Cornell Medicine

Stephen Liu
Lombardi Comprehensive Cancer Center, Georgetown University

Shirish Gadgeel
Henry Ford Health System

Balazs Halmos
Montefiore Medical Center and Albert Einstein College of Medicine

Author for correspondence: Matthew Lee, mlee7@montefiore.org

Abstract: The recent advances in the field of molecular diagnostic techniques have led to the identification of targetable alterations, prompting a paradigm shift in the management of non-small cell lung cancer (NSCLC) and an era of precision oncology. Herein, the authors highlight the most clinically relevant oncogenic drivers other than *EGFR*, their management, and current advancements in treatment. The authors also examine the different challenges in resistance to targeted therapies and diagnostic dilemmas for each oncogenic driver and the future direction of NSCLC management.

Keywords: non-small cell lung cancer, targetable mutations/alterations, resistance mechanisms, diagnostic techniques, driver mutations

ISBNs: 9781009336130 (PB), 9781009336123 (OC)
ISSNs: 2634-7490 (online), 2634-7482 (print)

Contents

1 Introduction   1

2 *ALK* Gene Rearrangements   5

3 *ROS1* Gene Rearrangements   12

4 *RET* Gene Rearrangements   16

5 *MET* Alterations   21

6 *KRAS* Point Mutations   27

7 *B-RAF* Point Mutations   32

8 *NTRK1/2/3* Gene Fusions   39

9 *ERBB2 (HER2)* Mutations   43

10 Diagnostic Strategies   48

References   54

1 Introduction

Lung cancer remains the number one cause of cancer-related deaths in the US and worldwide and non-small cell lung cancer (NSCLC) accounts for over 80% of all lung cancer cases.[1, 2] The advances of molecular diagnostic techniques and identification of targetable alterations (Figures 1 and 2) have ushered in the era of precision oncology, with targeted therapies and immunotherapy contributing to a decline in mortality of patients with NSCLC.[3] This Element will highlight the most clinically relevant oncogenic drivers other than *EGFR* (Table 1), their management, and novel treatments for each. We will also describe resistance mechanisms (Figure 3) and the diagnostic strategies (Table 2 and Figure 4) needed to define mechanisms of treatment resistance.

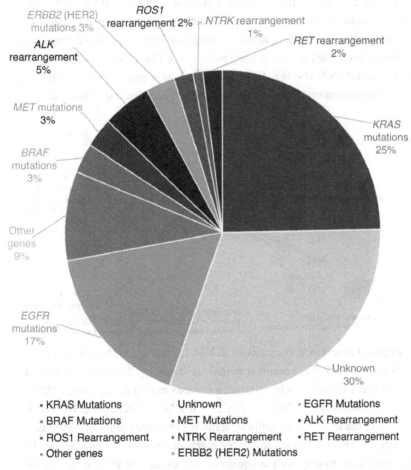

Figure 1 Non-small cell lung cancer oncogenic drivers

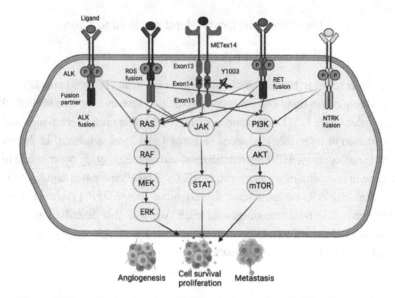

Figure 2 Signalling pathways and oncogenic targets of NSCLC. Important common signaling pathways of altered or mutated receptor and protein kinases that drive an increase in downstream activation of signaling proteins and transduction cascades. These include the signaling pathways of JAK-STAT, STAT, PI3K-AKT-mTOR, and RAS-RAF-MEK-KRK, and contribute to proliferation, migration, and survival mechanisms. Figure 2 was created with assistance with biorender.com

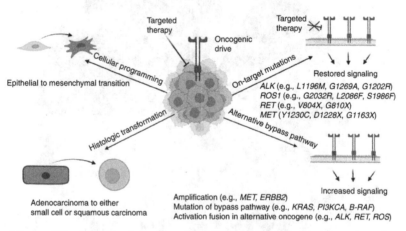

Figure 3 Resistance mechanisms in NSCLC that are harboring oncogenic driver mutations. The various acquired resistance mechanisms in oncogenic-driven NSCLC that include on-target mutations in *EGFR*, *ALK*, and *ROS1*, and off-target alterations in *RER*, *MET*, *KRAS*, *B-RAF*, *NTRK*, and *ERBB2* that both contribute to increased pathway signaling that leads to proliferation and metastasis. Other off-target resistance mechanisms depicted include histologic transformation to small cell or squamous cell carcinoma if the initial histology was adenocarcinoma along with epithelial to mesenchymal transition (EMT). Figure 3 was created with assistance with biorender.com

Table 1 Oncogenic drivers and their targeted therapies other than *EGFR*

Molecular oncogenic driver	ALK rearrangement	ROS1 rearrangement	RET rearrangement	MET exon 14	B-RAF V600E	KRAS G12C	NTRK1/2/3 fusions	ERBB2 alterations
First line	Alectinib (second gen)[22, 33] Brigatinib (second gen)[38] Crizotinib (first gen)[24] Ceritinib (second gen)[28] Lorlatinib[a] (third gen)[41]	Ceritinib (second gen)[28] Crizotinib (first gen)[71] Entrectinib (first gen)[78]	Cabozantinib[116, 117] Selpercatinib (second gen)[108] Pralsetinib (second gen)[123]	Capmatinib[b, 159] Crizotinib[b, 157] Tepotinib[c, 160]	Dabrafenib/trametinib[258, 260] Dabrafenib[258] Vemurafenib[264]	Sotorasib[205]	Entrectinib (first gen)[326] Larotrectinib (first gen)[322]	
Second line and beyond	Alectinib (second gen)[26] Brigatinib (second gen)[36, 37] Ceritinib (second gen)[28] Lorlatinib (third gen)[40]	Entrectinib (first gen)[108] Lorlatinib (third gen)[47]	Cabozantinib[116] Vandetanib[118]	No data	No data	No data	No data	No data
Emerging possible treatments	Ensartinib (second gen)[59] SAF-189[60]	Cabozantinib[82] Ensartinib[87]	BOS172738[131] TPX-0046[130]	Amivantamab[189] Cabozantinib[163]	Belvarafenib[301] Lifirafenib[305]	Adagrasib[207] BI1823911[215]	Repotrectinib[337] Selitrectinib[d]	Trastuzumab-deruxtecan (T-DxD)[367] Trastuzumab-emtansine (T-DM1)[363, 364]

Table 1 (cont.)

Molecular oncogenic driver	ALK rearrangement	ROS1 rearrangement	RET rearrangement	MET exon 14	B-RAF V600E	KRAS G12C	NTRK1/2/3 fusions	ERBB2 alterations
	TQ-B8301[61]	Repotrectinib[84]		Savolitinib[41]	PLEX8394[298, 300]	LY3537982[214]	Taletrectinib[300]	Poziotinib[362, d]
	TPX-0131[62]	Taletrectinib[86]		Telisotuzumab vedotin[a, 187]				Pyrotinib[358]
	NUV-655[63]			TPX-0022[184]				

[a] Treatment can also be used in oncogenic drivers including EGFR exon 19 deletions, L858R substitutions, T790M and C797S mutations, and EGFR exon 20 insertions, METex14 or MET amplification.

[b] METex14 and MET amplification inhibition

[c] METex14 inhibition only

[d] HER2, HER4, and EGFR exon 20 inhibitor

Abbreviations: gen, generation of targeted agent; METex14, MET exon 14, MET exon 14 skipping mutation

2 *ALK* Gene Rearrangements

2.1 Structure, Physiologic Functions, and Signaling Pathways

Anaplastic lymphoma kinase (ALK) is a member of the insulin receptor tyrosine kinase family[4] that has an extracellular ligand-binding domain, a transmembrane domain, and an intracellular tyrosine kinase domain.[5] The *ALK* gene was originally identified as a part of the nucleophosmin (*NPM1*)-*ALK* fusion gene in anaplastic large cell lymphomas by Stephen Morris et al. in 1994.[6] The ALK protein is activated by ligand binding that leads to downstream signaling via JAK-STAT, RAS-MAPK, and PI3K-mTOR.[7] Pleiotrophin, midkine, and small heparin-heparin-binding growth factors have been implicated as activating ligands for mammalian ALK.[8] Physiologic ALK signaling plays an important role in regulation of cell growth, differentiation, and transformation as well as development of the nervous system.[9, 10]

2.2 *ALK* Gene Rearrangements

ALK gene rearrangements are reported in 3–7% of NSCLC cases. They are more commonly described in patients who are young, are not, and have never been, smokers, and have adenocarcinoma.[11] The occurrence of de novo *ALK* rearrangements is mutually exclusive of other driver mutations; however, generally, there have been case reports of rare acquired *ALK* fusions along with *EGFR* mutations.[12, 13] The most common fusion partner of ALK is echinoderm microtubule-associated protein like-4 (*EML4*). *EML4-ALK* was first identified by Soda et al. and Rikova et al. in 2007.[14, 15] An inversion in chromosome 2p results in the fusion between the 3′ portion of *ALK* and the 5′ portion of *EML4*, creating the fusion gene that has constitutive tyrosine kinase activity.[14] Interestingly, *ALK* rearrangements can involve various breakpoints in the *EML4* gene or other non-*EML4* fusion partners, whereas the component of the *ALK* gene in the rearranged gene is constant.[16] Notably, the regulatory regions of the partner gene drive the initiation of the transcription of the ALK fusion protein.[17] The activation of the ALK kinase domain occurs via trans-autophosphorylation and homodimerization of ALK fusion proteins, a process that is also controlled by ALK fusion partners.[17] The constitutive activation of ALK fusion protein and downstream pathways promote cell proliferation and survival and generate antiapoptotic signals.[18] Based on the specific EML4 breakpoint, *EML4-ALK* fusions have been categorized into different variants and there are data to suggest that these variants may have prognostic and potentially predictive properties.[19]

2.3 Treatment

Crizotinib

Crizotinib is a potent ATP-competitive multikinase inhibitor (MKI) of ALK, c-Met, and ROS-1.[20] It was the first tyrosine kinase inhibitor (TKI) approved for the treatment of patients with advanced NSCLC that are harboring *ALK* gene rearrangement, after it showed a response rate (RR) of 57% in a phase I study (PROFILE 1001) that enrolled 82 previously treated patients.[21] These results were confirmed in the phase II trial, PROFILE 1005,[22] in previously treated patients with *ALK*-positive NSCLC. The overall response rate (ORR) was 59.8% and the median progression-free survival (PFS) was 8.1 months. Subsequently, crizotinib was studied in two phase III trials, PROFILE 1007 and PROFILE 1014, in second- and first-line settings, respectively. In PROFILE 1007, crizotinib was compared to docetaxel or pemetrexed in previously treated patients with *ALK*-positive NSCLC. Crizotinib showed a superior PFS (7.7 v 3.0 months, HR 0.49), RR (65 v 20%), and an improvement in quality of life.[23] In PROFILE 1014, first-line crizotinib was associated with longer median PFS (10.9 v 7.0 months, HR 0.45) as well as an improved RR (74 v 45%) compared to platinum plus pemetrexed.[24]

The most common adverse events (AEs) with crizotinib were vision disorders, diarrhea, and edema. The most common grade 3–4 AEs with crizotinib were elevations of aminotransferase levels and neutropenia. Grade 5 pneumonitis related to crizotinib treatment occurred in one patient who crossed over from the chemotherapy arm. Treatment discontinuation due to any AE occurred in 12% of patients treated with crizotinib.[24] Despite being the first ALK TKI to be approved, it is now rarely used since the introduction of more potent ALK TKIs.

Ceritinib

Ceritinib is a second-generation oral ALK inhibitor that inhibits the autophosphorylation of ALK.[16] It is FDA-approved in first- and second-line settings for the treatment of *ALK*-positive NSCLC. In the phase I trial ASCEND-1, ceritinib was investigated in an ALK inhibitor-naïve cohort (n = 83) and ALK inhibitor–pretreated cohort (n = 163). The RRs were 72 and 56% in the ALK-naïve and ALK-pretreated cohorts, respectively.[25]

In the ASCEND-2 phase II trial, ceritinib showed a median PFS of 5.7 months in patients treated with two or more lines of chemotherapy.[26] In the subsequent ASCEND-4 phase III trial, patients with treatment-naïve, *ALK*-positive NSCLC were randomized to receive ceritinib or platinum-based chemotherapy. Ceritinib demonstrated a superior median PFS (16.6 v 8.1

months, HR 0.55) and RR (73 v 27%).[27] In a second phase III trial, ASCEND-5, patients who had progressed on chemotherapy and/or crizotinib were random-ized to receive second-line treatment with ceritinib or chemotherapy. The median PFS was longer with ceritinib (5.4 v 1.6 months, HR 0.49).[28] The most common AEs in the ceritinib group were diarrhea, nausea, vomiting, and elevations in alanine aminotransferase.[28]

Alectinib

Alectinib is a second-generation ALK inhibitor. It is FDA-approved in first- and second-line (after progression on crizotinib) settings for patients with *ALK*-positive NSCLC. In a phase I/II trial, alectinib was investigated in ALK inhibitor-naïve patients with NSCLC and showed a RR of 93.5% (43/46 patients).[29] In another phase II trial in patients with *ALK*-positive NSCLC who had progressed on crizotinib, alectinib showed a RR of 48% and a median PFS of 8.1 months.[30] Thereafter, alectinib was compared to crizotinib in the first-line setting in two subsequent phase III trials.

In J-ALEX, Japanese patients with advanced *ALK*-positive NSCLC were randomized to receive alectinib or crizotinib. Alectinib was associated with prolonged median PFS (34.1 v 10.2 months, HR 0.37).[31] In an updated analysis, the five-year survival rates for patients in the alectinib and crizotinib arms were 60.85 and 64.11%, respectively.[32]

The ALEX trial was a phase III trial that randomized treatment-naïve Caucasian patients to receive alectinib or crizotinib, and demonstrated a superior median PFS (34.8 v 10.9 months, HR 0.43) and RR (82.9 v 75.5%) in the alectinib arm. Assessment of PFS by a blinded independent review committee showed better results with alectinib compared to crizotinib (25.7 v 10.4 months, HR 0.50).[19, 33] The five-year survival rate with alectinib was 62 versus 45% in patients treated with crizotinib;[34] however, this difference was not statistically significant. ALEX was also the first trial to prospectively evaluate the efficacy of these drugs against central nervous system (CNS) metastases. Alectinib was associated with a significantly prolonged time to CNS progression compared to crizotinib (p < 0.0001) and a higher CNS ORR of 85.7 versus 71.4%, respectively, in patients who received prior radiotherapy. The CNS ORR was 78.6 versus 40.0% in those who had not received prior radiotherapy in alectinib and crizotinib, respectively.[35]

Adverse events that occurred more frequently with alectinib compared to crizo-tinib were anemia (20 v 5%), myalgia (16 v 2%), increased serum bilirubin (15 v 1%), increased weight (10 v 0%), and photosensitivity (5 v 0%). Grade 3–5 AEs were more common with crizotinib (50 v 41%), and the most common grade 3–5 AEs in both groups were lab abnormalities. Adverse events leading to discontinuation were reported in 11% with alectinib and 13% with crizotinib.[33] Currently, in many treatment guidelines, alectinib is the preferred first-line treatment for patients with metastatic NSCLC that are harboring an *ALK* rearrangement.

Brigatinib

Brigatinib is a second-generation TKI that inhibits ALK fusion proteins. In the phase II ALTA trial, patients with *ALK*-positive NSCLC pretreated with crizotinib were randomized to receive two doses of brigatinib (90 mg daily and 180 mg daily with a 7-day lead-in at 90 mg). The RR was better with the higher dose of brigatinib (54 v 45%), as was the median PFS after two years of follow-up (16.7 v 9.2 months).[36, 37] In the phase III ALTA-1 L trial, brigatinib (180 mg daily with a 7-day lead-in at 90 mg) was compared to crizotinib in the first-line setting in patients with *ALK*-positive NSCLC. Brigatinib demonstrated superior PFS (24 v 11 months, HR 0.49) and RR (71 v 60%), and the intracranial ORR was 78% with brigatinib versus 26% with crizotinib. The intracranial PFS rate at two years was 48% with brigatinib versus 15% with crizotinib in patients with baseline CNS metastases, and 74 versus 67% in patients without baseline CNS metastases.[38, 39] Brigatinib is currently approved by the FDA in first- and second-line (after progression on crizotinib) settings.

Adverse events that occurred more frequently with brigatinib compared to crizotinib included an increased creatine kinase level (39 v 15%), cough (25 v 16%), hypertension (23 v 7%), and an increased lipase level (19 v 12%). Grade 3–5 AEs occurred in 61% with brigatinib and 55% with crizotinib. Pulmonary AEs occurred in 4% of patients treated with brigatinib, often characterized by early onset lung disease within 14 days of treatment initiation.[38] Due to acute pulmonary toxicity, patients start treatment at 90 mg daily for a week, and if no pulmonary events occur, the dose is increased to 180 mg daily. Brigatinib is considered in the first and subsequent lines of treatment for ALK fusion–positive NSCLC.

Lorlatinib

Lorlatinib is a third-generation ALK inhibitor specifically designed to target mutations in the ALK protein that causes resistance to crizotinib and next-generation TKIs. In preclinical studies, the drug was found to be effective against resistance mutations that may emerge after treatment with drugs such as alectinib, specifically G1202R.[16] In a phase II trial, patients were enrolled in six expansion cohorts to receive lorlatinib (EXP 1–6) based on *ALK* and *ROS-1* mutational status and previous therapy. An objective response was achieved in 90% (27/30) of the patients in the treatment-naïve EXP 1 cohort. In the EXP 2–5 cohorts, including those previously treated with TKIs (including crizotinib, ceritinib, and alectinib), objective responses were achieved in 47% of the patients.[40] Based on these results, the FDA granted accelerated approval to lorlatinib in patients with *ALK*-positive NSCLC who received two or more TKIs including crizotinib, or who progressed after first-line alectinib or ceritinib.

In the phase III CROWN trial, lorlatinib was compared in the first-line setting to crizotinib in patients with treatment-naïve *ALK*-positive NSCLC and demonstrated a superior PFS (78 v 39%, HR 0.28) and RR (76 v 58%).[41] Regarding CNS efficacy, the intracranial RR was 82% with lorlatinib versus 23% with crizotinib in patients with measurable brain disease. Moreover, 71% of the patients who received lorlatinib had an intracranial complete response (CR).

The most common AEs with lorlatinib were hyperlipidemia, edema, increased weight, peripheral neuropathy, and cognitive effects. Grade 3–4 AEs were more common with lorlatinib (mainly hyperlipidemia) compared to crizotinib (72 v 52%). Discontinuation of treatment because of AEs occurred in 7% with lorlatinib and 9% with crizotinib.[41] Lorlatinib has been shown to be an effective ALK inhibitor for both the first- and second-line treatments.

2.4 ALK Resistance Mechanisms

Acquired resistance is a significant clinical challenge in patients with *ALK*-positive NSCLC. Despite the high initial RR after crizotinib, patients relapse within one to two years.[42] ALK-acquired resistance is classified into *ALK*-dependent and *ALK*-independent mechanisms. In addition, there can be progression in sanctuary sites, specifically the CNS. Progression in the CNS is often due to restricted penetration of crizotinib through the blood–brain barrier. Fortunately, next-generation ALK inhibitors are very active against CNS metastases, but patients can experience tumor progression solely in the brain despite their effectiveness.

2.4.1 ALK-Dependent Resistance

ALK-dependent resistance occurs mainly due to mutations in the tyrosine kinase domain that decreases affinity for a TKI.[43, 44] *ALK*-resistant mutations rarely occur de novo and usually arise after treatment with ALK inhibitors.[45] The most common are the gatekeeper L1196 M and G1269A mutations found in 7 and 4% of crizotinib-resistant cases, respectively.[43] G1202R is a solvent-front mutation that confers resistance to crizotinib in 2% of the cases, but is more commonly seen after second-generation ALK inhibitors.[43] Other mutations, including C1156Y, G1202R, I1171T, S1206Y, and E1210K, are less common and found in around 2% of the cases.[43] Lorlatinib, a third-generation TKI, is a promising treatment option for patients who progressed on first- and second-generation TKIs due to resistant mutations. It showed activity in vitro against L1196 M- and G1202R-resistant mutations and in phase I/II trial in patients with known mutations after progressing on alectinib.[43, 46] In patients who progressed on second-generation TKIs, the RR to lorlatinib was reported to be higher among those with detected mutations in tissue sample and cell-free DNA (cfDNA) compared to others without mutations (62 v 32% based on cfDNA and 69 v 27% based on tissue samples).[47]

2.4.2 ALK-*Independent Resistance*

ALK-independent resistance can occur due to amplification of the *ALK* fusion gene or other downstream signaling pathways such as the insulin-like growth factor (IGF-1 R) and the epidermal growth factor receptor (EGFR).[48] Mutations in receptor tyrosine kinase (c-Kit) and mesenchymal-epithelial transition factor (MET) pathways have also been described as mechanisms of resistance to ALK inhibitors.[49] Epithelial to mesenchymal transition is another *ALK*-independent resistance mechanism that is defined pathologically as loss of cell-to-cell contact, enhancing cell motility and leading to cell detachment from parental epithelial tissue.[50, 51] This process allows cell migration, tumor invasion, and metastasis. No drug to date has been identified to address EMT-driven resistance.[43] Histologic transformation from adenocarcinoma to small cell carcinoma is another mechanism of resistance that has been described in *ALK*-positive NSCLC.[52]

2.5 Novel Strategies

Higher levels of PD-L1 expression have been described in up to 60% of *ALK*-positive NSCLC cases.[53] In preclinical models, anti-PD-1/PD-L1 antibodies showed promising results in *ALK*-positive NSCLC cell lines;[54] however, this has not translated to meaningful RRs in clinical settings.[55] In the phase III IMpower150 trial, patients with treatment-naïve metastatic non-squamous NSCLC, including those with *ALK*-positive tumors, were randomized to receive atezolizumab, carboplatin, and paclitaxel; bevacizumab, carboplatin, and paclitaxel; or atezolizumab, bevacizumab, carboplatin, and paclitaxel. Notably, patients with *EGFR* mutations or *ALK* aberrations had a longer PFS with atezolizumab and bevacizumab combined with chemotherapy as opposed to the combination without atezolizumab (9.7 v 6.1 months, HR 0.59).[56] The number of *ALK*-positive NSCLC patients in this cohort was very low. A novel approach to activating an antitumor response to *ALK*-positive NSCLC is required.

Further advances in the management of NSCLC are likely to occur through combination therapy, both for treatment-naïve patients and for patients previously treated with ALK inhibitors. Combining MET inhibitors with ALK inhibitors is a strategy currently being investigated in clinical trials based on preclinical data that demonstrated that cultured *ALK*-positive cells resistant to ALK inhibitors retained sensitivity to MET inhibitors.[57] Similarly, preclinical data have shown that SHP2 inhibitors may reverse resistance to ALK inhibitors and may also delay the development of resistance. Ongoing clinical trials are evaluating the combination of ALK and SHP2 inhibitors.

2.5.1 Adjuvant TKI Treatment

ALK inhibitors are being investigated in the adjuvant setting in patients with early-stage *ALK*-positive NSCLC in two clinical trials, ALCHEMIST (NCT02201992) and ALINA (NCT03456076). In the ALCHEMIST trial, patients with stage IB (tumor size $\geq$ 4 cm)–IIIA resected *ALK*-positive NSCLC are randomized to receive crizotinib versus observation after completion of chemotherapy and/or radiation. Crizotinib is administered for up to 24 months or until disease progression or unacceptable toxicities. The primary endpoint of this trial is overall survival (OS). Disease-free survival (DFS) and safety are secondary endpoints. ALINA is a phase III trial that is randomizing patients with stage IB (T $\geq$ 4 cm)–IIIA *ALK*-positive NSCLC at 4–12 weeks after resection to alectinib for 24 months (or until disease progression or unacceptable toxicities) versus four cycles of platinum-based chemotherapy.[58] The primary endpoint is DFS. Secondary endpoints are OS, safety, and pharmacokinetics.

2.5.2 Emerging Treatments for ALK Fusion/Rearrangement Inhibitors

Ensartinib

Ensartinib is a potent MKI that has shown activity against ALK, MET, and ROS1. In a recent phase III trial of treatment-naïve advanced *ALK*-positive NSCLC patients randomized to either ensartinib or crizotinib, the median PFS was significantly longer with ensartinib compared with crizotinib (25.8 v 12.7 months, p < 0.01).[59] The intracranial RR was 63.6% with ensartinib. The most common ensartinib treatment-related AEs (TRAEs) were rash, transaminitis, pruritus, nausea, constipation, edema, and anemia that were predominantly grade 2 or less. The most common grade 3 TRAE was rash in 11.2% of patients and managed with reducing and withholding the dose. The results suggest that ensartinib is a potential new first-line treatment option for patients with *ALK*-positive NSCLC.

SAF-189

SAF-189 is a selective ALK inhibitor with good penetration of the blood–brain barrier. In a preliminary analysis of a phase I/II study (NCT04237805) of previously treated patients with advanced *ALK*-positive NSCLC, SAF-189 treatment induced a partial response (PR) in 50% of patients.[60] Of those who had progressive disease after crizotinib or ceritinib, 48% demonstrated a PR with SAF-189, and those with brain metastasis demonstrated an equal 48% PR rate. The PFS data were immature at the time of the first data release and the trial is still ongoing but represents the harbinger of a potential ALK inhibitor with CNS activity for previously treated patients who had progressed after ALK inhibition.

TQ-B3101

TQ-B3101 is another MKI with ALK, ROS1, and MET inhibitory activity. It has been shown in a phase I study with patients who had progressed on kinase inhibitor therapy that the ORR was 62.5% in all cohorts and as high as 87.5% in the cohort receiving the highest dose.[61] Also, activity against CNS metastases was documented by an ORR of 62.5% in patients who had brain metastasis upon study entry. The most common grade 3 TRAE was neutropenia, transaminitis, and vomiting but was overall well tolerated. TQ-B3101 is currently being studied in a phase II trial with *ALK*-positive NSCLC patients who were previously treated with crizotinib (NCT04056572).

Novel Preclinical Treatments (TPX-0131 and NUV-655)

Two novel ALK inhibitors that have thus far shown preclinical activity are TPX-0131[62] and NUV-655.[63] Both compounds have been shown to have the ability to overcome many *ALK*-resistant mutations, including G1202R and L1196 M, and both have promising CNS-penetration potential. Taken altogether with early preclinical results, TPX-0131 and NUV-655 represent additional emerging ALK inhibitors with potential CNS penetrance ability.

3 *ROS1* Gene Rearrangements

3.1 Structure, Physiologic Functions, and Signaling Pathways

The *ROS1* gene is located on chromosome 6 and encodes an orphan tyrosine kinase of the insulin receptor family.[64] The ROS1 protein includes an intracellular tyrosine kinase domain, a transmembrane domain, and a large extracellular domain.[65] The normal function of ROS1 tyrosine kinase is currently unknown and no ligand for this receptor has been identified.[64] Biochemical studies of activated ROS have identified signaling to various downstream pathways such as PI3K/AKT, STAT3, VAV3, and MAPK.[64] There is about a 70% homology between ROS1 and ALK proteins, and some, but not all, ALK inhibitors inhibit ROS1 as well.[64]

3.2 *ROS1* Fusions

ROS1 rearrangements were first described in human glioblastoma cell lines involving 5′ end of the *FIG* (fused in glioblastoma) gene and 3′ end of *ROS1* through intrachromosomal deletion.[66] Subsequently, *ROS1* rearrangements were identified in multiple cancers including NSCLC,[15] cholangiocarcinoma,[67] gastric,[68] and ovarian cancers.[69] To date, nine *ROS1* fusion partners have been identified in NSCLC: *CCDC6, SDC4, EZR, TPM3, LRIG3, KDELR2, FIG,* and *SLC34A2* as well as the most frequent fusion partner, *CD47*.[70] *ROS1* rearrangements lead to a constitutively active tyrosine kinase, resulting in upregulation and activation of downstream pathways promoting cell survival and proliferation.[65] *ROS1*-rearranged NSCLC accounts for 1–2% of all cases.[65] NSCLC patients with *ROS1* rearrangements share many clinical features with patients that have *ALK* gene activation including younger age, absence of smoking history, and advanced stage disease at presentation.[65]

3.3 Treatment

Crizotinib

Crizotinib is a potent TKI of ALK, ROS1, and c-MET. It was the first TKI to receive FDA approval for the treatment of *ROS1*-rearranged NSCLC. In the expansion cohort of the phase I PROFILE 1001 trial, 50 patients with *ROS1*-rearranged metastatic NSCLC received crizotinib 250 mg twice daily. This trial showed a RR of 72%, median PFS of 19.2 months, and the updated median OS was 51.4 months.[71] OO-1201 is an open-label single-arm phase II trial in which 127 East Asian patients with *ROS1*-rearranged NSCLC received crizotinib, and had a RR of 71.7%. The median PFS was 10.2 months in patients with baseline CNS disease compared to 18.8 months in patients without baseline CNS disease.[72] EUCROSS is another single-arm phase II trial of 34 European patients with *ROS1*-rearranged NSCLC that showed a RR of 70% and median PFS of 20 months.[73] Despite reported efficacy, patients treated with crizotinib will eventually progress as drug resistance arises.[74] The crizotinib side effect profile in these trials is similar to its use in ALK fusion-positive trials in which the most common AEs include visual impairment, diarrhea, constipation, and peripheral edema and most common grade 3 TRAEs hypophosphatemia and neutropenia.

Ceritinib

Ceritinib is a second-generation TKI with activity against ALK and ROS1. Its efficacy was investigated in *ROS1*-rearranged NSCLC in a phase II study involving 30 crizotinib-naïve patients and demonstrated a RR of 67%, median PFS of 19.3 months, and intracranial ORR of 25%.[75] While ceritinib had promising results in patients with *ROS1*-rearranged NSCLC, its role in crizotinib-resistant cases remains limited due to lack of efficacy. Additionally, in the phase II trials, the incidence of AEs such as diarrhea, nausea, vomiting, and anorexia were higher with ceritinib than crizotinib.[76]

Entrectinib

Entrectinib is an MKI against ROS1, ALK, and NTRK with the ability to cross the blood–brain barrier.[77] Based on the pooled analysis of the STARTRK-1, STARTRK-2, and ALKA-372–001 trials, entrectinib was granted an accelerated FDA approval for the treatment of patients with *ROS1*-rearranged NSCLC.[78] In these trials, 53 patients with *ROS1*-rearranged advanced NSCLC were enrolled, 68% had received at least one prior line of therapy excluding ROS1 inhibitors. Patients received entrectinib at a dose of at least 600 mg once daily. The RR was 77% in the overall population, 74% in patients with baseline CNS disease, and 80% in those without CNS disease; and median PFS was 19 months, 13.6 months, and 26.3 months, respectively. The intracranial ORR was 55% and the degree of response in these trials was not different between patients with different ROS1 partners.[77, 79] The common side effects of entrectinib include dysgeusia, fatigue, dizziness, constipation, and nausea, and the most common grade 3 or more AEs were weight gain, anemia, and fatigue.

Lorlatinib

Lorlatinib is a selective ALK and ROS1 TKI with activity against some kinases with crizotinib-resistance mutations.[76] In an open label, single-arm phase I/II trial, 69 patients with *ROS1*-rearranged NSCLC received lorlatinib, 30% of which were TKI-naïve, 58% post-crizotinib, and 12% post one or two non-crizotinib TKIs. The RR in the overall population was 62%. Patients who were TKI-naïve had higher RR and PFS compared to patients who had progressed on crizotinib (62 v 35% and 21.0 v 8.5 months, respectively). Further analysis revealed that lorlatinib was unable to overcome G2032 R, the most common acquired *ROS1* mutation.[80] Intracranial RR was 64% in TKI-naïve patients and 50% in post-crizotinib patients.[80] The common TRAEs were hypercholesteremia, hypertriglyceridemia, edema, peripheral neuropathy, and cognitive effects. Similarly, the most common grade 3 or more TRAEs were also hypercholesteremia, hypertriglyceridemia, lipase elevation, and weight gain.

3.4 Resistance Mechanisms

Resistance mechanisms in *ROS1*-rearranged NSCLC can be divided into *ROS1*-dependent and -independent mechanisms. In *ROS1*-dependent mechanisms, mutations in the ROS1 kinase domain confer resistance to TKIs such as crizotinib and lorlatinib.[74] Lin et al. analyzed samples of 42 patients post-crizotinib and 28 patients post-lorlatinib, detecting ROS1 kinase domain mutations in 38% and 46%, respectively.[81] The most common mutation was G2032 R, detected in approximately a third of the cases. Additional mutations included S1986 F (2.4%) and D2033 N (2.4%) in post-crizotinib cases; and G2032 R/L2086 F (3.6%), G2032 R/S1986 F/L2086 F (3.6%), L2086 F (3.6%), and S1986 F/L2000 V (3.6%) in post-lorlatinib cases. This study also identified *ROS1*-independent resistance mechanisms such as *KRAS* amplification (4%), *KRAS* G12C mutation (4%), *MET* amplification (4%), *MAP2K1* mutation (4%), and *NRAS* mutation (4%).[81]

3.5 Future Direction

Resistance mutations post-TKI pose a major challenge in the treatment of *ROS1*-rearranged NSCLC. Lorlatinib showed promising efficacy in crizotinib-treated patients but failed against G2032 R, the most common resistant mutation with clinical results previously shown. Cabozantinib, a multi-kinase TKI with activity against RET, MET, VEGFR, and ROS1, has shown preclinical and clinical activity against crizotinib- and lorlatinib-resistant mutations including G2032 R, D2033 N, and L2086F.[82]

Repotrectinib

Repotrectinib (TPX-0005) is a TKI with activity against ALK, NTRK, and ROS1. In preclinical studies, repotrectinib showed activity against *ROS1* G2032 R and D2033 N mutations.[83] In the TRIDENT-1 phase I/II study, 39 patients with *ROS1*- and *NTRK*-positive NSCLC patients were treated with repotrectinib. The study included six expansion cohorts enrolling treatment-naïve and treated patients. The RR were 86%, 40%, 67%, and 40% in cohorts of TKI-naïve (prior platinum and immunotherapy), TKI- and platinum-pretreated, one prior TKI-pretreated, and two prior TKI-pretreated patients, respectively.[84] The TRIDENT-1 trial is currently enrolling globally, and results are awaited. Based on available results, the FDA has granted breakthrough designation for repotrectinib for patients with either treatment-naïve or previously treated *ROS1* positive NSCLC.

Taletrectinib

Taletrectinib is a selective ROS1 and NTRK inhibitor. Two previous phase I trials of NSCLC patients with *ROS1* fusions that received first-line taletrectinib had an ORR of 66.7% with a median PFS of 29.1 months from the US and Japan.[85] Preliminary results of an ongoing phase II trial TRUST (NCT04395677) in Chinese NSCLC patients with ROS1 fusions demonstrated an ORR among the crizotinib-naïve patients was 100%.[86] However, 82% of the patients had TRAEs that include transaminase elevation, neutropenia, nausea, vomiting, and diarrhea, and 13.6% were grade 3 or more, including fatigue, neutropenia, and transaminases.

Ensartinib

Ensartinib is an MKI that has activity against ROS1, ALK, MET, and NTRK and was examined in a phase II trial of Chinese patients with *ROS1*-positive NSCLC that had been previously treated with chemotherapy (NCT03608007).[87] Preliminary results showed an ORR of 27% with median PFS of 4.6 months, a median OS was not estimable. The trial also demonstrated intracranial responses with ensartinib after three of the four patients with brain metastases had intracranial disease control. The most common TRAEs were elevated transaminases and rash with grade 3 or more TRAEs at 25.4%.

4 *RET* Gene Rearrangements

4.1 Structure, Physiologic Functions, and Signaling Pathways

The *RET* (rearranged during transfection) gene was first discovered when NIH/3T3 cells were transfected with human lymphoma DNA, creating a rearranged oncogene.[88] The *RET* gene is located on chromosome 10 (10q11.2) and encodes for a transmembrane tyrosine kinase receptor that binds with a family of GDNF (glial cell line-derived neurotrophic factor) ligands that include NRTN (neurturin), ARTN (artemin), and PSPN (persephin) and one of four GDNF family of co-receptors.[89] After a ligand binds at one of the main docking sites (pY1062 or pY1096), dimerization and cross-autophosphorylation of the RET receptor's intracellular tyrosine kinase domains occurs. This then results in the activation of downstream pathways JAK/STAT, RAS/MAPK/ERK, and PI3K/AKT.[90–92] The downstream effects of these pathways are important for hematopoietic stem cell growth and embryogenesis of the urinary tract and enteric nervous system.[90–94] Moreover, another important role is that *RET* is also expressed normally in thyroid C-cells, and thus when mutated can has a role thyroid carcinoma pathogenesis.[95]

4.2 Clinical Disease States

A wide variety of *RET* alterations have been discovered comprising of substitutions, deletions, amplifications, and gene fusions.[96] These alterations occurring at the somatic level include *RET* fusions or *RET* mutations in malignancies such as medullary thyroid carcinoma (MTC) in up to 75% of cases, papillary thyroid carcinoma (PTC) in 5–10%, or NSCLC in up to 1–3%.[97–101] *RET* alterations can also occur in the germline to underlie multiple endocrine neoplasia 2 (MEN2), Hirschsprung's disease, or congenital defects of the kidney and urinary tract.[97, 102]

The majority of NSCLC with *RET* rearrangements are found in adenocarcinomas that often present with more advanced disease, as evidenced by up to 77% of patients presenting with stages III or IV and up to 45% developing brain metastases during the course of their disease.[103–105] Moreover, it has been reported that NSCLC patients with *RET* rearrangement are more associated with females, non-smokers, Asian ethnicity, and an age group of less than 60 years old compared to wild-type *RET* NSCLC patients.[105, 106] Nevertheless, a recent report has shown that there is no significant difference in either PFS or OS by *RET* status in patients treated with standard therapy prior to the advent of selective *RET* inhibitors.[107] Interestingly, patients with *RET*-altered NSCLC were also seen to have a lower response to immunotherapy with lower PD-L1 expression and tumor mutation burden (TMB),[105–109] which warrants further research and exploration if there are clinical implications.

4.3 *RET* Fusions

RET fusion proteins undergo ligand-independent dimerization and constitutive activation that leads to signal transduction in downstream pathways. To date, there are at least 13 *RET* fusion partners, with the most common upstream fusion partners in NSCLC being *KIF5B* (Kinesin-1 heavy chain) variants (70–90%) followed by *CCDC6* (10–25%) and the rest including *NCOA4, TRIM33, ZNF4, ERCC1, HTR4,* and *CLIP1* (~18%).[110–112] Irrespective of their fusion partners, *RET* fusions lead to the formation of a chimeric protein that includes the coiled-coil domain of their partner gene and the RET intracellular kinase domain leading to a ligand-independent activation and increased RET expression.[110–113]

4.4 Treatments

The first treatments for *RET* fusions that were developed were MKI with activity against RET, VEGFR2, MET, c-Kit, B-RAF, and EGFR. Examples of early MKIs used for *RET* fusions included cabozantinib, vandetanib, sunitinib, and lenvatinib.[105, 114–118] However, due to the numerous off-target toxicities that included hypertension, renal vascular injury, heart failure, and hand-foot syndrome, rates of dose reduction were as high as 73% and have fallen out of favor currently.[119–121]

Selpercatinib

To overcome the limitations of MKIs, highly selective RET TKIs have limited affinity for VEGFR2, and other kinases when tested in both wild-type and mutated *RET* patients. In 2018, selpercatinib (LOXO-292) was one of the first highly selective RET TKIs to receive the FDA approval for metastatic NSCLC patients with *RET* fusions based on the phase I/II LIBRETTO-001 trial (NCT03157128). It exhibited an ORR of 70% in patients previously treated with cisplatinum and 88% in treatment-naïve patients. The overall median PFS was 18.4 months,[108] with results not dependent on the type of previous treatment received. Selpercatinib was well tolerated, with only a 1.7% discontinuation rate, mainly grade 1–2 TRAEs with transaminitis, diarrhea, hypertension, and dry mouth, and only limited grade 3 or higher TRAEs with tumor lysis syndrome and increased aspartate aminotransferase.[108]

Pralsetinib

Pralsetinib (BLU-667) is another highly selective RET inhibitor with activity in both wild-type and mutated *RET* (*V804 L/M, M918 T, CCDC6*).[122] The FDA granted approval of pralsetinib for patients with metastatic NSCLC that are harboring *RET* fusions based on the phase I/II ARROW trial (NCT03037385) in patients with *RET* mutated MTC, NSCLC, and other advanced solid tumors. The results from this trial showed an ORR of 57% and 70% in 87 previously treated patients and treatment-naïve patients, respectively. The combined cohorts showed an ORR of 61%.[123] The majority of TRAEs were grade 1–2 and the most common treatment-related grade 3 or higher AEs were neutropenia (18%), hypertension (11%), and anemia (10%), with treatment-related discontinuation in 6%.[123] Other side effects include transaminitis, thrombocytopenia, and increase in creatinine and alkaline phosphatase along with pneumonia, pneumonitis, hemorrhagic events, tumor lysis syndrome, and risk of impaired wound healing.

Both selpercatinib and pralsetinib displayed up to 90% intracranial tumor responses.[108, 123] Results in the LIBRETTO-001 trial showed that of their 11 patients with CNS metastases, 2 had intracranial CRs and 8 had PRs,[108] and ARROW trial resulted with 7 of 9 patients demonstrating measurable shrinkage of brain metastases and no new CNS metastases.[123] Thus, not only are these two targeted agents safe and effective but they also display high CNS activity and have become important treatment options in metastatic NSCLC patients.

4.5 Resistance

The initial response to RET TKI therapy is relatively uniform, but invariably resistance is acquired over time. Mutations that confer resistance occur most commonly at the *RET* gatekeeper site or the solvent front area of the kinase.[122]

The most common mutations are *V804 L/M/E* that subsequently lead to steric hindrance and decreased binding of the TKIs to the ATP-binding pocket. This results in the MKIs having not only a lower efficacy but also a higher IC_{50} (half-maximal inhibitory concentration) values for each MKI.[122] The selective RET TKIs pralsetinib and selpercatinib have proven to be effective against these gatekeeper mutations and overcome the limitations of the MKIs. However, with selective pressure and continued usage of pralsetinib and selpercatinib, secondary resistance mutations develop mainly at the solvent front. These mutations include *RET* G810 R/S/C/V that also contribute to binding hindrance along with *KRAS* and off-target mechanisms such as bypass pathway activations (e.g., ERK and AKT) and *MET* amplification (15% of cases).[122, 124]

RET fusions themselves have also been implicated as mechanisms of acquired resistance in NSCLC that is driven by other oncogene mutations. Although in treatment-naïve NSCLC patients, oncogenic drivers such as *RET* fusions are generally considered mutually exclusive from other driver mutations, these same alterations can mediate acquired resistance to standard TKIs.[125] It has been reported that the highest rates of EGFR-TKI resistance from fusion genes are found in *RET* (38%), *ALK* (24%), *FGFR3* (14%), and *NTRK* (13%)[126] and that *RET* fusions can be found in 5% of biopsy material from osimertinib-resistant patients.[127] Rich et al. studied nearly 33,000 samples undergoing clinical plasma ctDNA testing at Guardant Health and identified 125 patients with NSCLC with RET fusions, including 17 with co-occurring EGFR mutations.[128] Specifically, only non-*RET-KIF5B* fusions contributed to the EGFR TKI resistance through MAPK pathway activation and other alterations.[128]

Given the role of *RET* fusions in EGFR TKI resistance, this has led to recent efforts studying the potential use of combining anti-EGFR and RET therapies. One report examined 12 NSCLC patients who had prior osimertinib and had either an *EGFR* exon 19 or L858 R mutation and an acquired *RET* fusion.[129] The patients then received a combination of osimertinib plus selpercatinib and five patients had a PR with a median duration of 7.4 months with the combination. Treatment was held in seven patients with disease progression and one patient for grade 2 pneumonitis. This demonstrated the feasibility of this combination and is pending future evaluation as an arm in the phase II ORCHARD trial (NCT03944772).

4.6 Future Directions

The *RET* oncogene has emerged quickly over the past decade as a crucial driver mutation for a variety of cancers. However, despite the advances in diagnostic capabilities of detecting fusion proteins, many areas need investigation, especially in terms of combination treatments and resistance to selective RET TKIs.

TPX-0046

New TKIs with novel chemical scaffolds are currently under investigation. Preliminary results of an investigational RET/SRC inhibitor, TPX-0046 from the ongoing phase I SWORD-1 trial (NCT04161391) in *RET*-altered NSCLC and MTC patients showed that four of the five previously untreated patients had tumor regressions with a duration of responses of at least 5 months.[130] In addition, of nine patients who were pretreated, three experienced tumor regressions. As reported in the early data, TPX-0046 seems to be well tolerated, with the most common TRAE being grade 1/2 dizziness, fatigue, constipation, and increase in alkaline phosphatase and lipase, with no grade 3 or higher TRAEs of transaminitis, hypertension, hemorrhagic effects, or cardiac or lung disease. Furthermore, TPX-0046 has been shown to have preclinical activity against solvent-front mutants such KIF5B-RET G810 R and represents a potential option for acquired resistance to selpercatinib or pralsetinib.[121]

BOS172738

BOS172738 is a highly selective RET and VEGFR2 inhibitor that has been shown in phase I results (NCT03780517) in *RET*-altered advanced solid tumors to have an ORR of 33% for NSCLC and 44% in MTC, with overall tolerable safety side effects of mostly grade 2 or higher, with some of the most common side effects being creatinine phosphokinase (CPK) increase, dyspnea, anemia, neutropenia, and diarrhea.[131] Other clinical drug candidates Pz-1 and NPA101.3 are other second-generation inhibitors of both VEGFR2 and RET are also under current investigation.[132]

5 *MET* Alterations

5.1 Structure, Physiologic Functions, and Signaling Pathways

The *MET* gene has emerged only recently as a key actionable oncogenic driver but was first discovered in the 1980s initially as a fusion protein (TPR-MET) on a human mutagenized osteosarcoma cell line that was exposed to the carcinogen MNNG (N-methyl-N'-nitro-N-nitrosoguanidine).[133] The *MET* gene is located on chromosome 7q21-q31 and encodes a tyrosine kinase receptor (c-MET) with extracellular, transmembrane, juxtamembrane, and kinase domains that are normally expressed by hepatocytes, neurons, and hematopoietic, epithelial, and endothelial cells.[134, 135] Binding of MET to its ligand HGF (hepatocyte growth factor) causes receptor homodimerization and autophosphorylation of intracellular tyrosine residues (Y1234 and Y1235) in its catalytic domain.[135] RET dimerization leads to the downstream activation of RAS/ERK/MAPK, PI3K/AKT, MTOR, WNT/β-catenin, JAK/STAT with activity in cell proliferation, migration, motility, EMT, embryonic development, angiogenesis, antiapoptotic signaling, and wound healing.[136–139]

Dysregulation in *MET* is present in 2–3% of all NSCLC and encompasses a wide variety of alterations. Examples include *MET* overexpression and rare *MET* fusion proteins but the most clinically relevant thus far being the primary oncogenic driver *MET* exon 14 skipping mutations (*METex14*) and *MET* amplification. Both of these types of alterations lead to activation of the MET pathways and have a role in acquired resistance to EGFR TKIs.[140]

5.2 *METex14* Alterations as Oncogenic Drivers

METex14 encodes the juxtamembrane domain of the MET receptor. It harbors the tyrosine 1003 (Y1003) binding site for the c-CBL E3 ubiquitin ligase that mediates protein degradation, but whose phosphorylation blocks caspase cleavage at aspartic acid 1002 (D1002) that occurs during apoptosis.[141, 142] Various alterations within exon 14 and its surrounding intronic regions include complete deletion of exon 14, insertions, indels at poly-pyrimidine tract (PPT), base substitutions, deletions at splice donor and acceptor sites, and point mutations at Y1003 or D1002. These all result in transcription disruption of METex14, leading to a shortened and activated c-MET.[143, 144]

MET exon 14 skipping mutations were first identified in 2005 in NSCLC and their incidence varies with histology.[145] It has been shown that 8–22% of the rare histologic subtype pulmonary sarcomatoid carcinomas contain *METex14* mutations that are found in 2–3% of adenocarcinoma and 1–2% of squamous cell carcinoma.[146–148] Patients with *METex14* also tend to be older, with the median age being 65–75 years old, frequently non-smokers, and more often female compared to those without *METex14*.[149–152] Furthermore, it has also been shown that those with *METex14* have a high frequency of metastases, with multifocal metastatic disease commonly in the lymph nodes, adrenal glands, pleural or pericardium, malignant effusions, bone, and brain.[153] *METex14* aberrations are rarely found with other oncogenic drivers and the prognosis of patients with *METex14*-positive tumors appears similar to lung cancers with other other driver mutations of kinases.[154, 155] Interestingly, *METex14* has been reported to overlap with *MET* amplification in 15–21% of *METex14* NSCLC patients and recently reported to be co-altered with *TP53* (42%), *MDM2* amplifications (34%), and CDK4 amplification (19%).[149, 156]

5.3 Treatments for *METex14* Skipping Mutations

METex14 splice site mutations that result in the *METex14* mutation have been demonstrated to be targetable in multiple clinical trials with mainly specific MET TKIs that prevent the phosphorylation process of tyrosine in the kinase domain.

Crizotinib

Crizotinib was one of the first multikinase MET inhibitors to be investigated as either first-line or subsequent line therapy option for metastatic NSCLC patients with *METex14* mutation. Clinical trials, such as the phase I/II trial PROFILE 1001 (NCT00585195), in patients with *METex14* advanced NSCLC treated with crizotinib had an ORR of 32% and PFS of 7.3 months,[157] and the phase II METROS trial (NCT 02499614) in previously treated NSCLC patients with advanced *MET* alterations showed an ORR of 20%, median PFS of 2.6 months, and OS of 3.8 months.[158] The most common TRAEs were vision disorders, nausea, vomiting, peripheral edema, diarrhea, transaminitis, and hypophosphatemia.

Capamtinib

Capmatinib is a selective MET inhibitor that has become the first approved agent for the treatment of *METex14* mutation in advanced NSCLC patients based on the results of the phase II GEOMETRY-trial (NCT02414139)d.[159] It was shown to have a benefit in both previously treated and treatment-naïve settings, with an ORR of 41% versus 68% and PFS of 5.4 months versus 12.4 months, respectively.[159] Overall, 13% of patients had TRAEs, with the most common including peripheral edema, nausea, vomiting, and an increase a serum creatinine level, along with 23% of patients requiring dose reductions and 11% discontinuing due to TRAEs.

Tepotinib

Tepotinib is another highly selective MET TKI that is approved for advanced NSCLC with *METex14* based on the phase II VISION trial (NCT02864992), resulting in an ORR of 46%, PFS of 8.5 months, and OS of 17.1 months in treatment-naïve and previously treated patients, respectively.[160] In contrast to crizotinib, tepotinib has greater CNS penetration, accounting for a CNS RR of 55% and PFS of 10.9 months in patients with CNS metastases holding promise as therapeutic for those with CNS metastases.[160] The most common TRAEs were peripheral edema, nausea, diarrhea, increase in serum creatinine, hypoalbuminemia and amylase/lipase. It was also reported that 28% of patients had grade 3 or higher with commonly peripheral edema (7%), leading to dose reduction in 33% of patients and 11% requiring discontinuation. One death was considered by investigators to be related to tepotinib with respiratory failure and interstitial lung disease.

Savolitnib

In a phase II trial (NCT02897479) of 61 patients with *METex14* NSCLC, savolitinib, a selective MET TKI, had an ORR of 47.5%, a PFS of 6.8 months, and an OS of 14.0 months in patients with advanced and metastatic NSCLC, including the aggressive pulmonary sarcomatoid carcinoma subtype.[161] The most common TRAEs were peripheral edema, nausea, vomiting, transaminitis, and hypoalbuminemia, with 14.3% of patients discontinuing due to TRAEs mainly due to liver injury and hypersensitivity. It has also recently been granted conditional approval in China for the treatment of patients with previously treated *METex14* NSCLC who progressed and are ineligible for chemotherapy, representing the first regulatory approval of savolitinib.

Cabozantinib

Cabozantinib is an example of an MKI that includes targets with MET, ROS1, VEGFR, RET, c-Kit, and FLT3. In a case series of 15 patients with *METex14* treated with either cabozantinib or crizotinib, 3 patients receiving cabozantinib had a PR and 1 patient had stable disease.[162] Currently, there is an ongoing phase II trial (NCT01639508) of cabozantinib in patients with RET/ROS1/ NTRK fusion-positive tumors or NSCLC with increased MET or AXL activity treated with cabozantinib. Another ongoing phase II trial, CABinMET (NCT03911193), is evaluating cabozantinib in previously treated or treatment-naïve NSCLC patients with *MET* amplification or *METex14*.[163]

5.4 Resistance Mechanisms

As MET TKIs have become widely adopted, resistance to these treatments has posed a significant challenge. Acquired on-target resistance is caused by various *MET* mutations, including MET kinase domain mutations with D1228X, Y1230X, H1094X, and G1163X.[164-167] These mutations affect the activity of type I MET TKIs such as crizotinib by disrupting the binding of the drugs to decrease affinity, cause steric hindrance, or reduce dephosphorylation, and has been reported to be present in up to 35% of resistance cases.[166] Other on-target resistance mutations in L1195 and F1200 residues have been implicated in resistance to type II MET TKIs such as cabozantinib.[168, 169] Off-target mechanisms comprise of 45% of resistance cases and include bypass pathways (e.g., PI3K, MEK) and concurrent oncogenic drivers such as *KRAS, EGFR, HER3*, and *B-RAF* amplification.[166, 170, 171]

Dual inhibition of MET and EGFR/ERBB2 both in vitro and in vivo may overcome resistance in cells that are harboring *METex14* mutations.[172] Sequential treatment with structurally different MET TKIs (type I or type II TKIs) was less effective, resulting in PRs in two out of six patients. One patient with an acquired crizotinib (type I TKI) resistance *MET Y1230C* mutation was then switched to merestinib (type II TKI) and another patient with amplification of *METex14* treated with glesatinib (type II TKI) was switched to crizotinib (type I TKI).[173] These results suggests that there is the potential of clinical response by switching to different structural MET TKIs. However, in two other cases when a type I MET TKI was switched to a type II MET TKI there was no response.[173]

5.5 *MET* Amplification

5.5.1 Role of MET *Amplification as a Primary Oncogene*

Increased *MET* gene copy number occurs either via focal amplification or through polysomy or genome duplication.[155, 174-176] De novo *MET* amplification has been reported in 1–5% of NSCLC with a higher frequency of 5–32% in pulmonary sarcomatoid histology subtype.[139, 148, 152, 177] High-level de novo *MET* amplification (*MET* to CEP7 ratio >5) tends to be mutually exclusive with other major drivers except for *METex14*, while low or moderate levels (*MET* to CEP7 ratio of 1.8–5) can harbor other driver mutations, including *EGFR/KRAS/ALK* mutations.[152, 176] De novo *MET* amplification appears to be associated with poorer prognosis, with shorter OS in high *MET* amplified cases compared to low or negative *MET* amplified patients.[139, 152] *MET* amplification as an oncogene itself remains a poorly validated target in the frontline setting and future studies are needed in its use as a biomarker.

5.5.2 Role of MET Amplifications in Acquired TKI Resistance

While de novo *MET* amplifications occur infrequently, acquired secondary *MET* gene amplification has emerged as a relatively common resistance mechanisms in TKI-treated lung cancer subsets, most particularly in *EGFR*-mutated NSCLC. EGFR inhibitor resistance attributed to *MET* amplification has been reported in 50–60% with first-generation EGFR TKIs and as high as 15–25% in those who progress on a third-generation EGFR TKI.[173, 178–180] The proposed underlying mechanism is that blockade of the EGFR causes a shift toward the MET pathway with a subsequent increase in *MET* amplification as a bypass alternative pathway.[179, 180]

Acquired resistance mediated by *MET* amplification has also emerged as a potentially actionable target. A phase Ib/II trial (NCT01610336) for patients with previously treated, EGFR-mutant and *MET*-amplified NSCLC were treated with the combination of the MET inhibitor capmatinib and EGFR inhibitor gefitinib. The results revealed an ORR of 27% overall amongst the entire cohort but a more robust response in the highly amplified MET cohort (MET gene copy number >6) with an ORR of 47%.[181] As for the TRAEs observed with the combination of gefitinib and capmatinib, the most frequent events were nausea, peripheral edema, and rash and the most common grade 3 and 4 events were elevated amylase and lipase levels, seen in 6% of patients. Similarly, the combination of the MET inhibitor tepotinib with gefitinib versus standard platinum chemotherapy was evaluated in the INSIGHT trial, a randomized phase Ib/II in patients with EGFR-mutant NSCLC previously treated with an EGFR inhibitor with *MET* overexpression or amplification.[182] In the *MET*-amplified cohort, tepotinib plus gefitinib had a median OS of 37.3 months versus 13.1 months with chemotherapy with a highly significant unstratified HR of 0.08 (0.01–0.51)[182] and a PFS of 16.6 months versus 4.2 months, respectively, with an unstratified HR 0.13 (0.04–0.43).[182] Both results suggest that this combination may be more effective in the *MET*-amplified *EGFR*-mutated NSCLC rather than non-*MET*-amplified EGFR-mutated NSCLC. The most common TRAEs to tepotinib and gefinitib were diarrhea, rash, elevated amylase levels, and peripheral edema, and the most common grade 3 or 4 TRAEs were increased amylase and lipase. All of these studies showed higher ORR in the *MET*-amplified subgroup, adding further evidence that *MET* amplification might be a key marker as opposed to MET expression in this context.

As seen from the results from these previous trials, there are many different combinations with mixed results, highlighting the need for further clinical studies on the optimal combination and sequence in *EGFR* mutant NSCLC patients with secondary *MET* amplification.

5.6 Future Directions

TPX-0022

One of the new therapies is a novel selective MET type I TKI, TPX-002. TPX-0022 targets the SRC oncoprotein, a kinase in the MET pathway involved in the upregulation of HGF, and also inhibits the colony-stimulating factor 1/colony-stimulating factor 12 receptor (CSF1 R/CSF12 R), which is involved with tumor-associated macrophages (TAMs).[183] The overall effect is inhibition of anticancer immune responses and activation of immune cytotoxic T cells.[184] TPX-002 is currently undergoing a first-in-human phase I trial, SHIELD-1 (NCT03993873), in patients with *MET* alterations and advanced solid tumors including NSCLC, with preliminary results showing 50% of treatment-naïve patients having a PR and majority of TRAEs being grade 1 or 2 with dizziness, fatigue, and increase in lipase and amylase, with no reported grade 4 or 5 TRAEs.[185]

Telisotuzumab Vedotin

Telisotuzumab vedotin, is an antibody-drug conjugate (ADC) comprised of an anti-MET antibody (ABT-700) complexed with a tubulin polymerization inhibitor (auristatin E, MMAE). Once telisotuzumab vedotin binds to MET receptors on tumor cells, it is internalized via endocytosis and delivers MMAE, leading to apoptosis. Another effect of this targeted approach is that it limits resistance mechanisms related to intracellular signaling such as *MET* amplification in EGFR TKI resistance.[186] Clinically, telisotuzumab vedotin has been shown to have single-agent activity in *MET*-amplified tumors in phase I studies, with notable ORRs of 60–75%.[187] A phase Ib study (NCT02099058) explored the combination of telisotuzumab vedotin and erlotinib in previously TKI-treated *EGFR*-mutated NSCLC, with *MET* overexpression showing ORR of 34.5% and a median PFS of 5.9 months. The most common TRAEs were dermatitis acneiform, diarrhea, neuropathy, and hypoalbuminemia with the most common grade 3 or higher TRAE being pulmonary embolism. Currently, an ongoing phase II trial (NCT03539536) with telisotuzumab vedotin in previously treated *MET*-altered NSCLC is underway and represents an intriguing option to overcome resistance.[188]

Amivantamab

Amivantamab (JNJ-61186372) is an anti-EGFR-MET bispecific antibody that has demonstrated efficacy in patients with *EGFR* exon 20-mutated NSCLC in a phase I trial CHRYSALIS (NCT02609776) in both previously treated or treatment-naïve NSCLC with *EGFR* mutation and *MET* amplification and mutations. The FDA has already granted accelerated approval and breakthrough therapy designation to amivantamab for *EGFR* exon 20 insertion mutated NSCLC and now the focus has turned toward its *METex14* cohort (MET-2 cohort). Preliminary results from the trial demonstrated that 64% had a PR to therapy regardless of prior lines of therapy and had a median PFS of 8.3 months and median OS of 22.8 months.[189] The most common TRAEs were rash, paronychia, hypoalbuminemia, and peripheral edema related, with 16% having grade 3 or higher TRAEs. Amivantamab represents another option in a growing field of targeted therapies for *METex14*.

6 *KRAS* Point Mutations

6.1 Structure, Physiologic Functions, and Signaling Pathways

KRAS is a member of the RAS family that binds GDP in its inactive state and GTP when active. RAS-K is a membrane-anchored protein by means of a fatty acid moiety covalently bound to a cysteine at the C-terminal end of the molecule. KRAS has two switch regions, switch-I and switch-II, that bind other effector and regulator proteins.[190] KRAS activates intracellular downstream pathways via hydrolysis of GTP to GDP, a process that transforms KRAS from an active to an inactive state.[191] The function of KRAS is regulated by guanine nucleotide exchange factors (GEFs) and GTPase activating proteins (GAPs). GEFs, such as SOS (son of sevenless), control the transformation of KRAS from the inactive (GDP-bound) to the active (GTP-bound) state, whereas GAPs, such as NF1, control active (GTP-bound) to inactive (GDP-bound) transformation.[192] KRAS regulates cellular proliferation through the activation of downstream pathways such as MAPK (RAF/MEK/ERK) and PI3K (PI3K/AKT/mTOR).[193]

6.2 *KRAS* Mutation Types

KRAS is one of the most mutated oncogenes in solid and hematological malignancies. Mutations in *KRAS* are frequently detected in lung (25%), pancreatic (90%), colon (35–50%), endometrial, biliary, and ovarian cancers.[194] Mutations in *KRAS* genes typically occur in major hotspots that affect the ability to hydrolyze GTP to GDP such as codons 12 (G12), 13 (G13), and 61 (Q61). Almost all pathogenic mutations are missense gain-of-function mutations resulting in insensitivity of mutated *KRAS* to GAP and thus increased levels of the GTP-bound active form of the protein, resulting in constitutive activation of the KRAS signaling pathway. This eventually leads to activation of downstream signaling proteins, such as MAPK and PI3K, promoting cell proliferation, cell survival, and metastatic potential.[193] Mutations in G12 and G13 occur in the GTPase domain of the protein, whereas Q61 mutations occur in the switch regions and interferes with NF1's ability to bind to KRAS and regulate its activity.[193] Mutations in codon 12 (G12) result from the exchange of glycine with another amino acid, such as G12C, G12D, and G12 V mutations.[195] G12 D and G12 V are very common in pancreatic cancer and can be found in 90% of the cases, G12 D mutation is the most common mutation in colon cancer, and G12C is detected in 13% of lung adenocarcinoma and 3% of colon cancer cases.[196]

6.3 Targeting *KRAS* Mutations

Decades of drug development failed to produce a therapeutic that successfully targeted RAS proteins.[197, 198] Initial attempts to target this molecule were focused on the direct inhibition of KRAS, which proved to be difficult due to its small size and shallow surface. Moreover, direct inhibition of KRAS had failed due to its high picomolar affinity to GTP and the lack of other hydrophobic pockets for drug binding.[196] Thereafter, researchers moved on to inhibit KRAS indirectly by targeting its post-translational processing. Before activation, RAS proteins undergo several post-translational modifications to mediate localization at the cell membrane, including farnesylation, geranylgeranylation, and palmitoylation, utilizing multiple enzymes such as farnesyltransferase (FTase), RAS-converting enzyme (RCE1), and isoprenylcysteine carboxyl methyltransferase (ICMT).[191] Inhibitors for these enzymes were developed and showed promising preclinical results; however, they failed in clinical studies, either due to side effects or lack of antitumor activity.[196] Afterward, efforts were directed to target KRAS downstream pathways MAPK and PI3K. MEK inhibitor monotherapy (trametinib) failed to show clinical benefit in a phase II study involving *KRAS*-mutated NSCLC patients.[199] Similarly, combination of an MEK inhibitor, selumetinib, and docetaxel did not demonstrate clinical benefit compared to docetaxel alone in patients with *KRAS*-mutated NSCLC previously treated with platinum-based chemotherapy. In 2013, Shokat et al. pronounced that the cysteine residue in G12C-mutant *KRAS* allows for the covalent and irreversible binding of compounds.[200] These findings led to the development of *KRAS* G12C inhibitors that resulted in the first successful targeting of mutant RAS protein activity.

6.3.1 KRAS *G12C* Inhibitors

Sotorasib

Sotorasib (AMG510) is an irreversible and highly selective inhibitor of G12C-mutated *KRAS* that binds allosterically to the switch-II pocket of the protein, trapping it in the inactive GDP-bound (OFF) state.[201] In preclinical studies, AMG510 showed durable tumor responses.[202] In clinical studies, sotorasib was evaluated in a phase I multicenter open label trial that enrolled 129 patients with pretreated NSCLC. Sotorasib showed an ORR of 35.5% at the target dose of 960 mg daily, with a median PFS of 6.3 months.[203] In the CodeBreaK-100 single-arm phase II trial, sotorasib was administered orally at a dose of 960 mg daily to 126 patients with previously treated advanced *KRAS* G12C-mutated NSCLC. In 124 patients, an objective response was achieved in 46 patients (37.1%), including 42 (33.9%) with PR and 4 (3.2%) with CR. Disease control rate (DCR) was around 80% (100 patients). Median PFS was 6.8 months and median OS was 12.5 months. An exploratory analysis demonstrated a lower ORR in patients with concomitant *KEAP1* mutations (ORR 20%) and higher ORR in patients with concomitant *STK11* mutations (ORR 40%).[204] The most common AEs were diarrhea, increase in the alanine aminotransferase levels, and fatigue.[205] Based on these results, the FDA granted sotorasib accelerated approval for patients with advanced *KRAS* G12C-mutated NSCLC who have received at least one prior line of therapy. CodeBreaK-200 (NCT04303780) is a phase III trial that is currently enrolling to evaluate sotorasib against docetaxel in second-line treatment of metastatic NSCLC.

Adagrasib

Adagrasib (MRTX849) is a potent irreversible inhibitor that binds covalently to cysteine in G12C-mutated *KRAS* in its inactive GDP-bound (OFF) state.[206] In KRYSTAL-1, a phase I/II open label multiple expansion cohort trial, 79 patients with unresectable or metastatic solid tumors were enrolled and had an ORR of 45%. The recommended phase II dose was 600 mg twice daily. The most commonly reported AEs were fatigue, increased LFT, QT prolongation, anemia, nausea, and vomiting. Treatment discontinuation due to AEs was reported in 4.5% of the patients.[207] The FDA has granted breakthrough designation for adagrasib for the treatment of previously treated *KRAS* G12C-mutated-positive NSCLC.

6.3.2 Resistance Mechanisms

Preclinical and clinical studies have started to reveal some of the resistance mechanisms that affect KRAS inhibitors. In vitro, 142 cell clones (Ba/F3) were developed that are resistant to either sotorasib or adagrasib. Koga et al. described 12 different *KRAS* secondary mutations in 124 (87%) of these clones. Interestingly, some mutations (G13D, A59S, A59 T, R68 M) confer resistance to sotorasib and not adagrasib, and vice versa (Q99 L).[208]

In the clinical setting, Tanaka et al. described a patient who developed resistance after treatment with adagrasib.[209] The patient had 10 emerging mutations affecting RAS-MAPK pathways, and three new *KRAS* mutations (G13D, G12 V, and Y69D). The switch pocket mutation Y69D was described to impair the binding of not only adagrasib but also sotorasib to *KRAS* G12C.[209] Awad et al. described a cohort of 38 patients treated with adagrasib, 27 patients with NSCLC, 10 with colorectal cancer, and 1 with appendiceal cancer.[210] Putative mechanisms of resistance were detected in 45% of the cohort (n=17), with 18% (n=7) carrying multiple cooccurring mutations. The resistance mechanisms described in this study included secondary *KRAS* mutations (G12D/R/V/W, G13D, Q61H, R68S, H95D/R/Q, Y96 C), high amplification of *KRAS* G12C allele, and acquired bypass mechanisms of resistance such as *MET* amplification; activating mutations in *NRAS, B-RAF, MAP2K1,* and *RET*; oncogenic fusions involving *ALK, RET, B-RAF, RAF1,* and *FGFR3*; and loss-of-function mutations in *NF1* and *PTEN*. Two patients with lung adenocarcinoma were found to have histologic transformation to squamous cell carcinoma without any other mechanism of resistance.[210]

6.4 Immune Checkpoint Inhibitors

Jeanson et al. investigated the efficacy of single-agent immune checkpoint inhibitors in patients with *KRAS*-mutated NSCLC and showed a numerically higher, but not statistically significant, ORR in patients with *KRAS*-mutated NSCLC compared to *KRAS* wild-type NSCLC (18.7 v 14.4%). Recent data suggest that concomitant mutations of other oncogenes can affect the immunogenic profile and response to immune-checkpoint inhibitors (ICIs) in *KRAS*-mutated NSCLC.[211] STK11 mutation reduces the efficacy of ICIs (ORR 7.4%) by reducing the expression of PD-L1, as well as increasing neutrophil recruitment and reducing the number of T-cells via production of pro-inflammatory cytokines. Patients with both *KRAS* and *KEAP1* mutations had significantly shorter OS (HR 1.96; $p \leq 0.001$) due to having lower PD-L1 levels and fewer T-cells in the tumor microenvironment.[212] Subgroup analysis of KEYNOTE-189 showed similar efficacy of pembrolizumab in combination with chemotherapy in patients with KRAS-mutated NSCLC compared to the overall study population (ORR 40.7%, median PFS 9 months, and median OS 21 months).[213] Additionally, there are studies evaluating immune checkpoint inhibitors and/or chemotherapy in combination with KRAS G12C inhibitors.

6.5 Future Directions

Building on the success achieved with sotorasib and adagrasib, additional KRAS G12C inhibitors are being developed and evaluated in preclinical and clinical studies. LY3537982 is a KRAS G12C inhibitor that showed encouraging preclinical results and will be evaluated in a phase I trial (NCT04956640).[214] BI1823911 is another compound that showed potent antitumor activity in preclinical studies. It is being evaluated in combination with a SOS1 inhibitor (BI1701963, NCT04973163).[215] Additionally, GDC-6036 and D-1553 are two inhibitors that are being evaluated in separate clinical trials as monotherapy or in combination with other agents in patients with advanced solid tumor that is harboring *KRAS* G12C mutations.[196] RM-032 has a novel mechanism of action as it inhibits KRAS G12C by forming a covalent bond with the protein in its active (ON) state and cyclophilin A (CypA). Preclinical studies showed encouraging results that seem to outperform KRAS G12C (OFF) inhibitors.[216] Other treatment modalities that target KRAS directly regardless of the presence of mutations are available and currently under evaluation, such as vaccines, adoptive T-cell therapy, proteolysis-targeted chimeras (PROTACS), and CRISPR/Cas9 reagents.

Furthermore, acquired resistance to KRAS G12C inhibitors is a major challenge in treating patients harboring this mutation. Bypassing or overcoming this obstacle is an area of unmet need and multiple strategies are currently being studied to achieve this goal. One strategy is combination therapy of KRAS (G12C) inhibitors with compounds targeting upstream or downstream pathways. SHP2 is an upstream target that alters the ability of KRAS to transform between its two states (active and inactive), inhibition of SHP2 can enhance the efficacy of KRAS(G12C) inhibitors.[217] Currently, TNO155 and RMC-4630, two SHP2 inhibitors, are being evaluated in clinical trials in combination with adagrasib (NCT04330664) and sotorasib (NCT04185883), respectively. Another strategy is inhibition of downstream pathways, such as mTOR and MEK. In vivo, adagrasib showed potent activity when combined with mTOR inhibitor, vistusertib.[218] CodeBreaK1 (NCT04185883) is a phase I study evaluating sotorasib alone or in combination with other anticancer therapies including MEK inhibitor trametinib.

7 *B-RAF* Point Mutations

7.1 Structure, Physiologic Functions, and Signaling Pathways

B-RAF is one of the isoforms of RAF that codes for a serine/threonine kinase protein that transduces downstream signals via the RAS-RAF-MEK-ERK in the MAPK pathway. RAF kinases are stimulated through the activation of RAS via a GDP-GTP exchange factor called SOS factor that promotes RAF dimerization. This then initiates the MEK/ERK signaling cascade that contributes to cellular growth, differentiation, proliferation, and survival.[219] This pathway is regulated by multilevel negative feedback loops that include direct inhibitory phosphorylation of B-RAF and SOS factors from ERK activation along with the induction of inhibitory proteins NF1, Spry (sprouty), and DUSP (dual-specificity phosphatases), all of which ultimately results in both decreased upstream and downstream signaling.[220–224] These regulatory features provide a basis for understanding not only the normal physiologic balance of this pathway but also with implications for B-RAF oncogenic drivers in terms of therapy responses and resistance.[224, 225]

The *B-RAF* gene is located on chromosome 7 (7q34). The protein contains three highly conserved domains (CR1, CR2, and CR3), each with their own unique properties.[222, 226] CR1 contains the RAS-binding domain with the ATP-phosphate-binding loop (P-loop), CR2 contains the 14–3–3 binding site, and C3 located on the C-terminal encompasses the kinase domain regulated by phosphorylation.[227, 228] In the inactive B-RAF kinase state, hydrophobic interactions and a-helices form stabilizing bonds between the P-loop, activation segment, and the Asp-Phe-Gly (DFG) motif.[229] Phosphorylation of these activating loops destabilize the a-helices and hydrophobic interactions and make the catalytic clefts available for binding and activation.[228]

7.2 B-RAF Alterations

Mutations in *B-RAF* were first identified in 2002 as somatic missense and substitution point mutations within exon 15, which is involved with the activation segment of the kinase domain and within exon 11, which is involved with the P-loop.[230–232] Since then, a wide variety of *B-RAF* mutations have been detected in patients with melanoma (50–60%), papillary thyroid cancer (30–50%), colon cancer (10%), and NSCLC (1–3%).[232, 233] *B-RAF* mutations are categorized broadly into three classes based on their kinase activity and RAS-dependence.

Class I *B-RAF* mutations produce constitutively active B-RAF kinase monomers that result in high kinase activity and activated ERK but are independent of upstream RAS signaling and do not require dimerization for activation of MAPK signaling.[233] One of the most common and best-studied *B-RAF* mutant proteins is B-RAF V600E that is derived from a transversion mutation at T1799A on exon 15, causing a substitution of a glutamic acid (E) for valine amino acid (V) at codon 600 in the kinase domain.[234] Additionally, class I *B-RAF* mutations include other amino-acid substitutions in position 600 with the same effect as V600E such as V600K or V600D.[220]

The predominant *B-RAF* mutation in lung cancer is B-RAF V600E but with improvements in diagnostic capabilities with next-generation sequencing (NGS) and cfDNA, recent studies have now suggested that 30% or up to as high as 50–80% of B-RAF mutations in NSCLC are non-V600 B-RAF class II constitutively active dimers or class III heterodimer mutations.[219, 228, 233, 235–239] This contrasts with melanoma in which B-RAF V600E is the predominant protein of *B-RAF* mutations.[238]

Class II mutations are also RAS independent but form B-RAF mutant dimers that strongly activate the MEK-ERK pathway, causing the inhibition of the negative feedback loop of upstream signaling and low levels of RAS-GTP.[233, 240] These mutations are present in the activation segment (L597Q/R/S/V) or P-loop (G464A/E/V/R, G469V/R).[234, 240, 241] Class III mutations are RAS-dependent with enhanced binding to C-RAF and RAS as heterodimers with mutant B-RAF and wild-type C-RAF and other wild-type RAFs. These alterations may also cooccur with NF1 tumor suppressor deletions or RAS activation mutations with a dependency on upstream signaling, high RAS-GTP levels, and low or no kinase activity.[240] Class III mutations are present in the P-loop (G466A/E), DFG motif (D594 N/G/A, G596D/R), and catalytic loop (N581S/I).[219, 228, 233]

In terms of the clinicopathological features of *B-RAF* mutations in NSCLC, they are generally mutually exclusive from other driver mutations such as *EGFR* or *ALK*.[230, 234] Specifically, *B-RAF* V600E is associated with adenocarcinoma with more aggressive histopathology with micropapillary features,[242] shorter DFS, and OS rates[243] along with lower response to platinum-based chemotherapy compared with patients without *B-RAF* mutations.[244] In addition, *B-RAF* V600E mutated patients have been associated with females, non-smokers, and have a lower incidence in Asians (1.3%) than in Caucasians (3%).[230, 234]

Non-V600 mutations (class II and III) are also present mainly in adenocarcinomas but also in squamous cell carcinoma with an association with males and smokers, more likely to have brain metastases, shorter PFS on chemotherapy, and lower OS compared to *B-RAF* V600E class I mutations.[237, 240, 241, 243, 245] However, further studies are needed if NSCLC patients with non-V600 variants are a distinct prognostic group, as in colorectal cancer.[246]

B-RAF fusions are even rarer than B-RAF mutations and only found in 0.2% of NSCLC patients and 2.8% of *B-RAF* mutations.[238] Common *B-RAF* fusion partners include *ARMC10, AGK, DOCK4,* and *TRIM24*[238, 247], and *B-RAF* fusions cooccurred with gene mutations of *TP53, CDKN2A, EGFR,* and *CDKN2B*.[247] *B-RAF* fusions have predominantly been found in lung adenocarcinoma females, with a low median TMB of 3.8–4.8 muts/Mb,[247, 248] but further studies are needed on the prognostic outcomes of these patients. Although rare, *B-RAF* fusions play an important role in acquired resistance to EGFR TKIs and are more frequently associated with resistance cases rather than de novo primary oncogenic drivers.[249]

7.3 Treatments

Initial studies regarding targeting *B-RAF* mutations focused on inhibition of RAF monomers such as vemurafenib and dabrafenib in patients with metastatic melanoma that are harboring B-RAF V600E. However, it was shown that the combination of MEK inhibitors such as dabrafenib and trametinib had superior outcomes compared to monotherapy with a B-RAF inhibitor alone in melanoma patients with fewer toxicities.[250, 251] This is explained by the previously mentioned negative feedback loops that are present in the RAS-RAF-MEK-ERK pathway. When RAF is targeted alone in *B-RAF* V600E mutants, this results in both a decrease in ERK reactivation but also a decrease in the negative feedback loop that normally inhibits the wild-type RAS or RAF activation.[223, 252, 253] This leads to a paradoxical activation of wild-type RAS and RAF isoforms such as CRAF, causing ongoing MAPK pathway activation.[254, 255] Furthermore, this paradoxical pathway activation has also led to increased skin toxicities such as cutaneous squamous cell carcinoma, especially when type I B-RAF inhibitors such as vemurafenib and dabrafenib are applied as monotherapies in metastatic melanoma patients with *B-RAF* V600E mutations.[256, 257] The concept of dual B-RAF-MEK inhibition has also been applied in patients with metastatic NSCLC with a *B-RAF* V600E mutation.

Dabrafenib

In an open-label phase II trial BRF113928 (NCT01336634), patients were treated with either dabrafenib and trametinib or monotherapy dabrafenib. The results of the trial demonstrated that dabrafenib as a single agent in the second-line setting had an ORR of only 27% but an even larger treatment effect was seen with the combination of trametinib and dabrafenib with an ORR of 63% and 61% in previously treated and treatment-naïve cohorts, respectively.[245, 258] Updated analysis on the trial revealed that the PFS was 10.2 months and an OS of 18.2 months in the combination arm compared to a PFS of 5.5 months and an OS of 12.7 months in dabrafenib alone.[259, 260] The most common TRAEs (>20%) in the combination arm included pyrexia, nausea, vomiting, fatigue, diarrhea, edema, rash, cough, and dyspnea, with 69% having grade 3 or higher events, permanent discontinuation in 12%, and dose in a reduction in 35% of patients.[245, 258] Based on this trial, the FDA approved this combination in 2017 and is now the standard of care in patients with metastatic *B-RAF* V600E-mutated NSCLC in either the first- or subsequent-line setting.[261]

Vemurafenib

Another B-RAF inhibitor, vemurafenib, approved in combination with cobimetinib (a MEK inhibitor) for advanced or metastatic *B-RAF* V600-mutated melanoma,[262] has been studied as monotherapy in *B-RAF* V600-mutated unresectable or metastatic NSCLC patients in a phase II study.[263] In the 62 patients with NSCLC with *B-RAF* V600 mutation, the median OS was 15.4 months, median PFS was 6.5 months, and the ORR in both the treated and previously treated cohorts was 37.1%, with no difference based on prior treatments. Similarly, another recent trial of 96 patients with *B-RAF* V600-mutated NSCLC and treated with monotherapy vemurafenib, the ORR was 44.8%, the median PFS was 5.2 months, and median OS was 10 months, the most frequent TRAEs were asthenia, decreased appetite, acneiform dermatitis, and nausea/diarrhea.[264] This demonstrated promising results and a safety profile similar to melanoma studies and may be another possible option. However, there are no published studies of the combination of vemurafenib and cobimetinib in *B-RAF* V600-mutated NSCLC, but there is an ongoing phase II multicenter trial (NAUTIKA1, NCT04302025) that will help examine its efficacy in this cohort. It will involve resectable stage II–III NSCLC patients with a wide variety of oncogenic drivers, including *B-RAF* V600, who will then be treated with neoadjuvant vemurafenib plus cobimetinib for eight weeks and then adjuvant chemotherapy, and up to two years of vemurafenib and cobimetinib.

Therapy for *B-RAF* Class II and III Mutations in Lung Cancer

As for *B-RAF* non-V600 variants with class II and III mutations, it has been challenging to treat these variants due to their heterogenous functionality and exclusion in clinical trials. There are no approved treatments and monotherapy B-RAF inhibitors have shown to be not efficacious in these types of variants. For example, in a multicenter study that included both *B-RAF* V600E and non-V600 mutations, only one patient (17%) with a *B-RAF* non-V600 had a clinical benefit from monotherapy of vemurafenib with PR compared to an ORR of 54%

in the V600E cohort.[265] In addition, patients with *B-RAF* non-V600 mutations had a worse PFS of 1.5 versus 9.3 months and an OS of only 11.8 versus 25.3 months compared to patients with *B-RAF* V600E-mutated NSCLC.[265] Furthermore, in the AcSe vemurafenib trial, the *B-RAF* non-V600 cohort had an ORR of 0%, median PFS of 1.8 months, and median OS of 5.2 months and was stopped after it met the trial's stopping criterion.[264]

Monotherapy with the MEK inhibitor trametinib has also been studied in patients with *B-RAF* non-V600 mutations. A multicenter phase II trial of patients with melanomas with *B-RAF* non-V600 mutations demonstrated significant clinical activity, with three of the nine patients having objective responses or 33%, and two other patients with stable disease and a median PFS of 7.3 months.[266] However, an NCI-MATCH (National Cancer Institute Molecular Analysis for Therapy Choice) trial with multiple phase II tumor agnostic arms examined a total of 32 patients with *B-RAF* non-V600 variants and *B-RAF* fusion across multiple different cancers that included NSCLC (28%) showed a PR of only 3%, and 10 patients with stable disease, a median PFS of 1.8 months, and an OS of 5.7 months. It concluded that trametinib had relatively low activity and the primary endpoint was not met.[267]

Combination dual inhibition with B-RAF and MEK inhibitors have demonstrated promising results in *B-RAF* non-V600 variants. In an in vitro and in vivo study that examined two metastatic melanoma samples with *B-RAF* L597S, it was found that single-agent dabraenib or trametinib was insufficient to shrink the tumors; only with dual inhibition with dabrafenib and trametinib was there a response.[268] This was also demonstrated both in vitro[269] and in case reports of patients with *B-RAF* non-V600-mutated NSCLC that responded to combinations such as dabrafenib and trametinib.[270–273] However, the responses of *B-RAF* non-V600-mutated variants may also be influenced on other concomitant genetic alterations such as *KRAS* mutations and the type of mutations such as B-RAF G469V, which have been shown in-vitro showing higher resistant to combination therapy.[273]

Immunnotherapy

Immunotherapy has been studied in retrospective studies in which patients with both *B-RAF* V600- and *B-RAF* non-V600-mutated NSCLC had ORRs of 25% and 33%, respectively, but there was no difference in median OS or PFS between the two groups.[274] Another retrospective study involving immunotherapy in previously treated *B-RAF*-mutated NSCLC also reported similar results, with an ORR of 28%, median PFS of 3.1 months, and an OS of 13.6 months.[275] These retrospective studies may indicate not only similar activity of immunotherapy regardless of the type of *B-RAF* mutation in NSCLC but also that efficacy of immunotherapy suggests a higher sensitivity rate in this oncogenic driver compared to other drivers.[275–277] However, its utility as either monotherapy or combination and timing still requires research and requires further studies.

7.4 Resistance

Resistance is mediated by many different mechanisms that are broadly categorized as either primary or secondary resistance to B-RAF inhibitors but have mainly been studied. *B-RAF* mutations have also been implicated as causes of acquired secondary resistance, especially involving EGFR TKIs in NSCLC. However, overall, there is very limited data on both primary and secondary resistance of *B-RAF*-mutated NSCLC and further studies are needed. The majority of research for primary intrinsic resistance to B-RAF inhibition is focused on melanoma, and mechanisms include loss of *PTEN*, mutations in *NF1, MEK* and *CDK4* mutations, and cyclin D1 amplifications.[278–282]

Secondary resistance to B-RAF/MEK inhibition has also been studied, mainly in melanoma, with a majority due to alterations in the MAPK pathway and ERK reactivation causing reactivation in PI3K-AKT-mTOR, EGFR, and other alternative bypass pathways.[219, 225, 283–285]

In terms of NSCLC with *B-RAF* V600E-mutatated NSCLC, there is a paucity of data in terms of resistance, and studies are mainly from case reports/series of patients that had acquired resistance to B-RAF/MEK inhibitors with mutations such as *MEK1 K57N, NRAS Q61R/K*, and *KRAS Q61R/G12D/V*.[286–289]

7.4.1 Role in Acquired Resistance to EGFR TKIs

Activating *B-RAF* mutations are usually mutually exclusive with activating *EGFR* mutations, but *B-RAF* mutations or fusions may arise during the development of EGFR TKI resistance in 1–2% of cases, resulting in the reactivation of MAPK signaling.[226, 239, 290] It has been shown that patients with acquired EGFR TKI resistance from *B-RAF* fusions retain either the primary *EGFR* mutations or TKI-resistant EGFR T790 M or C797S.[247, 290] However, management for these cases has been thus far based on case reports and preclinical studies. For example, osimertinib resistance caused by *B-RAF* V600E can be overcome to some degree by triplet sequential therapy with dabrafenib, trametinib, and osimertinib[291–294] or in acquired *B-RAF* fusions with osimertinib and trametinib.[239, 249, 295, 296] Moreover, an in vitro study has shown a pan-RAF inhibitor (LY3009120) used as monotherapy blocked the growth of mutant *EGFR* cell lines with *B-RAF* fusion.[239] However, larger clinical studies are needed to verify these results and this novel therapeutic strategy.

7.5 Future Directions

B-RAF mutations are composed of a heterogeneous group of distinct classes and clinical features that poses ongoing treatment and diagnostic challenges. Further research is still needed, especially in *B-RAF* non-V600 variants, as much of the treatment targets only class I mutations.

Pan-RAF Inhibitors

There is growing promise and potential in pan-RAF inhibitors (e.g., LY3009120, PLX8394, PLX7904, belvarafenib) that have been added to avoid the paradoxical ERK/MAPK pathway reactivation.[277, 297–300] They specifically inhibit ERK signaling and disrupt *B-RAF* mutant dimers that are commonly found with B-RAF fusions and splice variants that are a major cause of acquired resistance to B-RAF inhibitors and have utility in both V600 and non-V600 mutants.[277, 297–299] These pan-RAF inhibitors are currently undergoing phase I/II trials in advanced or metastatic *B-RAF*-mutated NSCLC as single-agent therapies: PLX8394 (NCT02328712), LY3009120 (NCT02014116), and belvarafenib (NCT02405065, NCT03118817).[301]

ERK Inhibitor

ERK inhibitors are currently being studied as another approach to inhibit downstream targets since ERK reactivation is a common mechanism of acquired resistance to B-RAF and MEK inhibitors. In phase I trials involving advanced or metastatic solid tumors with *B-RAF* V600 mutations, ERK inhibitors have shown acceptable safety profiles but varied clinical responses. ERK inhibitor GDC-0094 has an ORR of 33%,[302] but in MK-8353[303] and Ulixertinib[304] (BVD-523), they only have responses in melanoma patients with an ORR of 20% and 12%, respectively. These may not be effective as single agents for inhibition of B-RAF but may need to be combined with other agents that block further upstream signaling.

RAF and EGFR Inhibitor

Lifirafenib (BGB-283) concurrently targets both EGFR and B-RAF. In a phase I trial (NCT02610361), patients with either *B-RAF* or *KRAS/NRAS* mutations driving solid tumors had tolerated this medication, the most common grade 3 TRAEs were hypertension (17.6%) and fatigue (9.9%). One lung cancer patient was among the eight patients with *B-RAF* mutations with confirmed OR.[305]

8 *NTRK1/2/3* Gene Fusions

8.1 Structure, Physiologic Functions, and Signaling Pathways

In 1982, *NTRK* was initially discovered as an oncogene in a colon cancer sample during gene transfer assays and was initially called *OncD*.[306] After fully mapping the *OncD* locus, it was found to be a fusion gene involved with *TRK (tropomyosin receptor kinase)* and *NTRK (neurotrophic receptor tyrosine kinase)*, first identified as the fusion product *TPM3-NTRK1*.[307] A total of three *NTRK* genes (*NTRK1, NTRK2,* and *NTRK3*) each encode a transmembrane receptor tyrosine kinase (TRKA, TRKB, TRKC), respectively. They were located on chromosomes 1q21-q22, 9q22.1 and 15q25.[308] The TRK receptors consist of an extracellular domain, transmembrane region, and tyrosine kinase domain that interact with ligands including NGF (nerve growth factor), BNDF (brain-derived neurotrophic factor), NT-3 (neurotrophin-3), and NT-4 (neurotrophin-4).[308] After ligand binding and receptor dimerization, the TRK receptor undergoes autophosphorylation of intracellular tyrosine residues located within the activation loop of the kinase domain, causing an activation of downstream pathways such as PI3K/AKT, RAS/MAPK, and PLCG, which are subsequently involved with synaptic transmission, neuronal development, differentiation, and survival.[310, 311]

8.2 Rearrangement and Fusions of NTRK1, NTRK2, and NTRK3

Rearrangements occur through various routes that include usually in-frame fusions such as *NTRK* gene fusing with a partner gene. There are over 80 gene partners that have been described, with the most common being ETV6 and TPM3. The majority of these fusions subsequently lead to overexpression of these TRK proteins and constitutive activation of the downstream pathways, causing proliferation and survival of cancer cells, suppression of E-cadherin expression, and enhancement of matrix metalloproteinase-2 (MMP-2).[312, 313] *NTRK* fusions have been rarely identified in common cancer types, such as in less than 1% of papillary thyroid cancer,[314] gliobastoma,[315] cholangiocarcinoma,[316] head and neck squamous cell carcinoma, and lung cancer,[309] but *NTRK3* fusions are dominant in over 90% of patients with rare cancer types such as secretory carcinoma, infantile fibrosarcoma, cellular mesoblastic nephromas, and mammary analogue secretory carcinoma.[310, 317]

An *NTRK1* gene rearrangement was first described in an NSCLC patient with a *TMP54-NTRK2* rearrangement.[318] The clinical significance of TRK fusions in NSCLC patients revealed that the majority are younger, with a median age at diagnosis of 47.6 years, and have never smoked, with a median pack year history of 0 (range, 0–58).[319] Furthermore, there was also an association of high TRKB and BDNF expression, with shorter OS and DFS along with a higher prevalence of nodal metastases and more advanced stages.[313, 320]

8.3 Treatments

NTRK fusion tumors are driven by NTRK tyrosine kinase for their proliferation and survival, and thus TKIs are the cornerstone treatment option for these mutations. The FDA approval of first-generation NTRK TKIs, larotrectinib (2018) and entrectinib (2019), were based on basket trials involving metastatic or unresectable cancers with NTRK fusions.[321]

Larotrectinib

Larotrectinib was one of the first TRK inhibitors that was found to be highly selective for TRKA, TRKB, and TRKC and was shown to have efficacy in a combined analysis of three phase I/II clinical trials (NCT02122913, NCT02637687, and NCT02576431). These trials included both adult and pediatric patients with TRK fusion-positive cancer and reported an ORR of 79%, PFS of 28.3 months, and OS of 44.4 months.[322–324] The most common TRAEs were fatigue, elevated transaminases, and cough of all grades, and with grade 3–4 AEs occurring in about 14% of patients with elevated transaminases, anemia, and neutropenia.[323]

Entrectinib

Entrectinib is a first-generation *NTRK* inhibitor that inhibits TRKA/B/C, ROS1, and ALK.[325] Entrectinib was studied in multiple clinical trials, including the phase I adult trials with ALKA-372–001 (EudraCT, 2012–000148–88) and STARTRK-1 (NCT02097810), and phase II basket trial STARTRK-2 (NCT02568267) that included *NTRK1/2/3, ROS1, or ALK*-rearranged positive cancers. In a pooled analysis of these three clinical trials with a total of 54 adults with ten different tumor types, the ORR was 69% in patients with NSCLC, the median OS was 14.9 months, and the median PFS was 14.9 months.[326, 327] Entrectinib has also been shown to penetrate the blood–brain barrier with efficacy in patients with brain metastases, resulting in improved median time to CNS disease progression.[326] The

ORR in a cohort of NTRK fusion-positive NSCLC patients with and without baseline brain metastasis was 67% in nine patients and 75% in four patients, respectively.[327] The most common AEs reported in over 20% of patients included fatigue, cognitive impairment, and gastrointestinal disorders, with other serious side effects consisting of hepatotoxicity, heart failure, prolonged QT, and neurotoxicity, with 4% requiring discontinuation due to TRAEs.[326, 327]

8.4 Resistance

Resistance to the first-generation NTRK inhibitors such as entrectinib and larotrectinib are either from acquired on-target or off-target resistance mechanisms. On-target resistance mechanisms involve mainly substitution mutations either at the hydrophilic solvent front (G595 R, G623 R), gatekeeper region (F589 L, F663 L, F617 L), or activation loop xDFG motif (G667 C, G696A) in the NTRK kinase domain.[321, 328, 329] The resistance mutations cause alterations in the conformations, leading to steric hindrance of drug binding or/and decreased ATP-binding affinity.[321] In an analysis of acquired resistance in the STARTRK-2 (NCT02568267) trial, it was reported that 34% of 29 paired samples had a newly acquired NTRK solvent front mutation at disease progression that was not present in the pretreatment sample.[330]

As for off-target resistance, similar to other oncogenic drivers, there have been reports of bypass pathways such as MAPK activation from MEK1 (MAP2K1) P124S mutation, *MET* amplification, activated IGF-1 R pathway, or other alterations such as an acquired *B-RAF* V600E or *KRAS* G12A/G12D mutations.[311, 321, 331]

8.5 Future Directions

To overcome resistance mechanisms, a new generation of NTRK inhibitors that have a higher affinity for the wild-type and mutant NTRK isoforms are currently being examined. The most promising of these include selitrectinib, repotrectinib, and taletrectinib.

Selitrectinib

Selitrectinib (LOXO-195) is a second-generation TRK inhibitor that has a similar chemical structure to larotrectinib but is more selective and displays activity against secondary resistance mutations at the solvent front and xDFG mutations.[332, 333] From the phase I/II study (NCT03215511, NCT03206931) of those who relapsed on prior TRK inhibitors such as larotrectinib and entrectinib, results report an ORR of 34% in the overall evaluable population in 10 of the 29 patients and an ORR of 45% in the cohort, with an acquired on-target *TRK* kinase mutation in 9 of the 20 patients.[334] However, three patients who were resistant due to TRK-independent mechanisms with bypass pathways did not respond to selitrectinib, highlighting the need for different approaches to off-target resistance mechanisms. The most frequent TRAEs were dizziness/ataxia, ataxia, nausea, vomiting, anemia, and gait disturbance.[334]

Repotrectinib

Repotrectinib (TPX-0005) is another second-generation NTRK inhibitor that also has activity with *ALK* and *ROS1* but has additionally been shown to overcome acquired resistance from larotrectinib- and entrectinib-harboring solvent front mutations (e.g., TRKA (G595 R), TRKB(G639 R), TRKC(G623 R)) and displaying in vitro the highest affinity for the NTRK mutant proteins compared to selitrectinib, entrectinib, and larotrectinib. Repotrectinib was the only treatment that was active against NTRK1 G595 R and F589 L.[335, 336] Repotrectinib is currently being examined in phase I/II trial TRIDENT-1 (NTC 03093116) in *NTRK1/2/3, ROS1,* and *ALK* fusion cancers. Preliminary data with repotrectinib from six NSCLC patients after TRK TKI treatment had a 50% ORR after salvage therapy.[337]

Taletrectinib

Taletrectinib (AB-106; DS-6051b) like repotrectinib is also an *ROS1* and *NTRK* kinase inhibitor but mainly has been studied in the *ROS1*-positive population. In a pooled analysis of two taletrectinib phase I studies from the US (NCT02279433) and Japan (NCT02675491), there were a total of 22 patients with *ROS1*-positive NSCLC that showed an ORR of 66.7%, and median PFS of 29.1 months in ROS1 TKI-naïve patients and 14.2 months for crizotinib refractory patients.[85] An ongoing phase II trial, TRUST (NCT04395677), is evaluating taletrectinib in *ROS1*-positive Chinese NSCLC patients, and preliminary results have shown an ORR among crizotinib-naïve patients of 90.5% and crizotinib previously treated patients of 43.8% and an intracranial ORR of 83.3%.[338] However, 81.8% had TRAEs that include transaminitis, nausea, vomiting, diarrhea, and neutropenia, and 13.6% required dose interruption.[338]

Combination Therapies with TRK TKIs

Combination therapies combining TKIs to TRK and other kinases have been examined in individual experiments but not in large clinical trials. One preclinical example of a xenograft model from a *CTRC-NTRK1* fusion-positive pancreatic cancer patient developed resistance to larotrectinib with an acquired *B-RAF* (V600E) and *KRAS* (G12D) mutation that resulted in significantly more suppression of tumor growth with triple therapy that included larotrectinib, dabrafenib, and trametinib compared to dabrafenib and trametinib alone. In a cholangiocarcinoma patient with an acquired *MET* gene amplification after selitrectinib treatment had tumor shrinkage at eight weeks and disease control by 44.5 months with disappearance of *NTRK* fusion and *MET* amplification by circulating free DNA testing from a combination of selitrectinib with crizotinib.[321] Given the response of combination treatment and the common convergence of *B-RAF* (V600E), *KRAS* (G12D), and *NTRK* fusions with MAPK pathway activation, the combination of selitrectinib and the MEK inhibitor trametinib was shown to be more effective than either single agent in suppressing activation of TRK and ERK in a selitrectinib-resistant model with *LMNA-NTRK*, *NTRK1* G595 R, and *KRAS* G12D mutations.[321]

9 *ERBB2 (HER2)* Mutations

9.1 Structure, Physiologic Functions, and Signaling Pathways

ERBB2 (HER2) is a transmembrane receptor encoded by the *ERBB2* gene on the long arm of chromosome 17 (17q12).[339] It is a member of the human epidermal growth factor receptor tyrosine kinase family along with EGFR, ERBB3, and ERBB4.[339] ERBB2 has neither a ligand nor ligand-binding domain, but is the preferred heterodimerization partner for the other three members of the EGFR family. Receptor activation leads to activation of downstream signaling pathways such as MAPK and PI3K.[340] This process ultimately leads to cellular proliferation, migration, and differentiation.[340]

9.2 *ERBB2* Alterations

ERBB2 alterations in NSCLC can occur in three mechanisms: protein overexpression, gene amplification, and point mutation. ERBB2 overexpression has been defined in most NSCLC studies as a score of 2+ or more on immunohistochemistry (IHC).[341] The incidence of ERBB2 overexpression in NSCLC is 2–38% and is most frequently found in well-differentiated pulmonary adenocarcinoma.[342] The prognostic significance of ERBB2 overexpression in NSCLC is controversial. Most recently, a meta-analysis that included more than 6,000 patients concluded that ERBB2 overexpression is a poor prognostic factor for patients with NSCLC.[343] *ERBB2* gene amplification is defined as an average ratio of the *ERBB2* gene copy number to the centromere of ≥ 2.0 on fluorescence in situ hybridization (FISH).[344]

ERBB2 amplification is reported in 3% of NSCLC cases without prior exposure to EGFR TKI and in 13% of those with prior EGFR therapy as a mechanism of resistance to EGFR TKI.[342] The correlation between ERBB2 amplification and overexpression is well described in breast cancer, however, it couldn't be confirmed in NSCLC.[342]

ERBB2 gene mutations constitutively activate the receptor leading to uncontrolled cell proliferation and have been determined to be driver mutations in NSCLC.[345] They have been reported in 2–4% of patients with NSCLC, most commonly in cases of adenocarcinoma in women, people who have never smoked, and people of Asian ethnicity.[346] The most common *ERBB2* mutation, accounting for 80–90% of the cases, is the insertion or duplication of the amino acids tyrosine, valine, methionine, and alanine (YVMA) at codon 776 (YVMA 776–779 ins) in exon 20.[347] *ERBB2* mutations have been described as mutually exclusive of other driver mutations; however, the European EUHER2 cohort reported five patients with concimitant *EGFR, ALK,* and *ROS1* alterations.[348] Moreover, the correlation of *ERBB2* mutation with gene amplification and protein overexpression in NSCLC is still unclear.[342]

9.3 Treatment

9.3.1 Multikinase Inhibitors

Afatinib

Afatinib is an irreversible pan-ERBB TKI. It was first evaluated in a phase II trial in patients with pretreated NSCLC that are harboring *EGFR* and *ERBB2* mutations. In patients with *ERBB2* mutations, afatinib demonstrated a DCR of 71% (5/7) and a median PFS of 17 weeks. The most common AEs were diarrhea and rash.[349] In the NICHE phase II trial, 13 patients with pretreated *ERBB2*-mutated NSCLC were enrolled to receive afatinib as monotherapy. The reported ORR and DCR were 7.7% and 53.8%, respectively. The median PFS and median OS were 3.7 months and 13 months, respectively.[350]

Dacomitinib

Dacomitinib is an irreversible pan-ERBB TKI that inhibits EGFR, ERBB2, and ERBB4. In a phase II trial, 26 patients with pretreated *ERBB2*-mutated NSCLC received dacomitinib and had an ORR of 12%. The median PFS and OS were 3 months and 9 months, respectively. The responses were observed in patients with non-YVMA (A775_G776 ins) mutations. The most common AEs were diarrhea and rash.[351]

Neratinib

Neratinib is another irreversible pan-EGFR TKI. In the SUMMIT phase II basket trial, 26 patients with pretreated *ERBB2*-mutated NSCLC were treated with neratinib and had an ORR of 3.8% (1/26). The PFS was 5.5 months. The most common AEs were diarrhea, nausea, and vomiting.[352] Neratinib was also investigated in a phase II trial in combination with temsirolimus, an mTOR inhibitor. The study enrolled 62 patients and showed an ORR of 19% in the combination arm and 0% in the monotherapy arm. Patients treated with the combination had more stomatitis (49 v 6%).[353]

9.3.2 Selective TKIs

Poziotinib

Poziotinib is an irreversible EGFR and ERBB2 inhibitor. It showed promising antitumor activity in preclinical and early phase clinical trials.[354] In a phase II trial that included patients with pretreated NSCLC that are harboring *EGFR* or *ERBB2* mutations, the ORR was 42% with median PFS of 5.6 months in patients with *ERBB2* mutations. The most common side effects were diarrhea (17%) and rash (58%).[355] In the multicenter phase II trial ZENITH20 (ongoing), 90 patients with pretreated *ERBB2*-mutated NSCLC received poziotinib. An interim analysis showed an ORR of 27.8% and a median PFS of 5.5 months. CNS-specific DCR and ORR were 100% and 28.6%, respectively. The most commonly reported TRAEs were rash, diarrhea, and mucositis.[356]

Pyrotinib

Pyrotinib is a pan-ERBB inhibitor that showed promising results in preclinical studies.[357] In a single-center phase II study including 15 patients with pretreated *ERBB2*-mutated NSCLC, the ORR was 53.3% (8/15) with a median PFS of 6.4 months.[358] In a confirmatory multicenter phase II trial, 60 patients with pre-treated *ERBB2*-mutated NSCLC were enrolled. The reported ORR was 30% with a median PFS of 6.9 months and OS of 14.4 months. The most frequent AEs were diarrhea (91.7%, grade 3 or higher 28.3%), elevated serum creatinine, and vomiting.[359]

9.3.3 Monoclonal Antibodies

Trastuzumab

Trastuzumab is a monoclonal antibody that binds to the extracellular-IV domain of ERBB2, preventing its dimerization and activation. The role of trastuzumab in NSCLC is limited.[357] In a retrospective analysis of 57 patients with pretreated

ERBB2-mutated NSCLC who received trastuzumab and chemotherapy, the ORR was 50% and the median PFS was 4.8 months.[348] In contrast, trastuzumab monotherapy failed to show an objective response in a phase II trial that included seven patients with pretreated *ERBB2*-mutated NSCLC.[360] In another phase II trial, 101 patients with untreated *ERBB2*-amplified or -overexpressed NSCLC were randomized to receive gemcitabine and cisplatin with or without trastuzumab. In the overall population, no difference in ORR or PFS was detected between two treatment arms (41 v 36%; 7 v 6.1 months). However, in IHC 3+ or FISH-positive cases (n = 12) the ORR was 83% and median PFS 8.5 months with trastuzumab plus chemotherapy. In the trastuzumab arm, three patients had >15% decrease in their left ventricle ejection fraction, a known toxicity of trastuzumab.[361]

Pertuzumab

Pertuzumab is another monoclonal antibody that blocks the ERBB2 dimerization domain, inhibiting its heterodimerization with other members of the EGFR family. In the phase IIa MyPathway basket trial, 30 patients with pretreated *ERBB2*-mutated or -positive NSCLC received trastuzumab and pertuzumab. The ORR was 21% and 13% in the two populations, respectively.[362]

9.3.4 Antibody-Drug Conjugates

Trastuzumab-Emtasine

Trastuzumab-emtansine (T-DM1) is an anti-ERBB2 ADC constituting of trastuzumab and the cytotoxic microtubule agent emtansine (DM1). T-DM1 is internalized into *ERBB2*-positive cells through receptor-mediated endocytosis where it releases DM1 after proteolysis via cellular lysosomes.[357] A phase II trial that evaluated T-DM1 monotherapy in 15 patients with *ERBB-2*-altered relapsed NSCLC was closed early due to limited efficacy.[363] Another phase II trial evaluated T-DM1 at the dose of 3.6 mg/kg intravenously and showed a median PFS of five months for patients with *ERBB2*-mutated NSCLC and ORR of 50%. For patients with *ERBB2*-amplified NSCLC, ORR was 55%. The majority of AEs were of grade 1–2, and included increased liver enzymes, thrombocytopenia, and nausea.[364]

Trastuzumab-Deruxtecan

Trastuzumab-deruxtecan (T-DxD) is a novel ERBB2-targeting ADC constituting of trastuzumab, an enzymatically cleavable peptide linker, and a topoisomerase I inhibitor (MAAA-1181). The chemotherapeutic molecule works by binding to and stabilizing topoisomerase I-DNA complexes, leading to DNA double-strand breaks and apoptosis.[357] T-DxD's stable design and high membrane permeability facilitate its diffusion across *ERBB2*-negative or -low conditions.[365] In vitro, it showed promising antitumor activity against T-DM1-resistant cells.[365] In a phase I trial, T-DxD was administered to 11 patients with relapsed *ERBB2*-mutated NSCLC. Reported ORR was 72.7% and median PFS was 11.3 months.[366] In the recently published phase II DESTINY-Lung01 trial, 91 patients with refractory *ERBB2*-mutated NSCLC treated at a dose of 6.4 mg/kg demonstrated an ORR of 55%. The median PFS was 8.2 months and median OS was 17.8 months. Grade 3 or higher AEs occurred in 46% of patients, the most commonly reported was neutropenia (19%). Drug-related interstitial lung disease occurred in 26% of the cohort, 75% of which were grade 1–2. However, four patients had grade 3 pulmonary toxicity and two patients died. Notably, responses were observed across different *ERBB2* mutations and were not dependent on *ERBB2* over-expression or amplification.[367]

9.4 Resistance

Most of the data we have on resistance mechanisms come from breast and gastric cancer; however, resistance mechanisms were also elucidated in NSCLC. *ERBB2*-independent resistance can occur due to activation of PI3K/AKT and RAS/MAPK pathways.[368] Secondary *ERBB2* mutations such as L755S and T789I were reported as *ERBB2*-dependent resistance mechanisms.[369] In a large retrospective study that included 66 patients with *ERBB2*-altered NSCLC treated with afatinib, NGS was performed on blood and tissue from nine patients after progression. *ERBB2* alterations were still detected in seven out of nine patients (78%). Secondary ERBB2 mutations were detected in three patients (p. G776delinsLC, Y772_A775dup, and amplification). *TP53* was the most frequently mutated gene in 44% of the patients, followed by *EGFR* (33%). Lastly, one patient had *NRAS* mutation, and another patient had no *ERBB2* alteration detected after progressing on afatinib.[370]

9.5 Combination Therapy and Future Directions

Treatment of patients with *ERBB2*-altered NSCLC has achieved promising results with monotherapy approaches and soon we expect that combination therapies of ADCs with TKIs and/or ICIs will change the landscape of *ERBB2*-altered NSCLC. Preclinical studies have provided evidence to support moving combination therapies into the clinical setting. Li et al. showed that the combination of T-DM1 and neratinib enhanced internalization and ubiquitination of ADC by the cells leading to higher antitumor activity.[371]

Robichaux et al. reported similar results after combining T-DM1 and pozio-tinib in *ERBB2*-mutated cell lines.[372] Moreover, T-DxD has been shown to increase tumor-infiltrating CD8+ T-cells and PD-L1 expression in breast cancer cells.[373] This finding led to the initiation of multiple clinical trials that evaluated the activity of ICIs in addition to T-DxD in patients with *ERBB2*-altered NSCLC, such as: the HUDSON (NCT03334617), DESTINY-Lung03 (NCT04686305), and KEYNOTE-797 (NCT04042701) trials

10 Diagnostic Strategies

The accuracy and reliability of diagnostic methods is essential in the manage-ment of NSCLC patients in order to identify predictive markers for therapy selection. The numerous diagnostic techniques include detecting alterations at the DNA level employing FISH or DNA-targeted NGS. Genetic analysis can also be done on serum samples to analyze for circulating tumor DNA (ctDNA). At the RNA level, diagnostic tests include reverse transcriptase polymerase chain reaction (RT-PCR) or RNA-based NGS. Protein analysis is done by IHC. Each diagnostic tool has its own advantages and limitations and how it is incorporated into testing algorithms has become an integral part in guiding treatment for each NSCLC patient (Table 2).

10.1 Tissue-Based

10.1.1 Immunohistochemistry

One of the most widely accessible and widespread diagnostic techniques is IHC. It is used in distinguishing both histologic subtypes of lung cancer patients and used mainly in identifying aberrant expression levels of fusion proteins by utilizing optimized primary antibodies that target specific regions of interest in the fusion protein.[374] Importantly, the success of this approach requires low-absent normal protein levels in tumors that lacked fusions. This has allowed IHC to be used as either a screening tool for rearrangements or as a surrogate marker for *ALK* rearrangements and, with limited specificity, for translocations of *RET, ROS1*, and *NTRK* that cause protein overexpression and often require confirmation with other molecular techniques.[374–382] IHC use in identifying oncogenic drivers in mutations such as in *EGFR* and *B-RAF* has been disap-pointing and not used in these situations.[374, 383–385] The emerging utility of *MET* IHC as a predictive biomarker for targeted MET therapy in *METex14* and *MET* amplification has yet to be widely validated and accepted in diagnostic practice due to the heterogeneity of MET IHC assessments and lack of stand-ardized cutoff points.[386–389] Lastly, there is growing interest in identifying

Table 2 Diagnostic platforms for NSCLC oncogenic drivers[a]

	IHC	FISH	RT-PCR	Tissue-based NGS (DNA, RNA)	Liquid biopsies (ctDNA)
Fusions and rearrangements:	✓[b]	✓		✓	✓
ALK					
ROS1					
RET					
NTRK			✓	✓	
Point mutations:				✓	✓
EGFR					
KRAS					
B-RAF					
MET					
Indels (insertions or deletions):	✓			✓	✓
EGFR exon 19 deletion					

[a] The most common alterations in NSCLC and the essential diagnostic methods to diagnose, screen, or confirm these oncogenic drivers.

[b] Requires FISH confirmation for *ROS1*, *RET*, and *NTRK* fusions/rearrangements and diagnosis cannot be based solely on IHC staining

✓ indicates the approved usage of a molecular diagnostic method for the specific alteration examined

Abbreviations: ctDNA, circulating tumor DNA; FISH, fluorescence in situ hybridization; IHC, immunohistochemistry; NGS, next-generation sequencing; RT-PCR, reverse transcriptase polymerase chain reaction

ERBB2 (HER2) mutations in NSCLC patients and like other cancers such as breast and gastric cancers. IHC has emerged as a key diagnostic strategy for HER2 overexpression and complements and sometimes replaces testing with FISH.[390, 391] This combination of IHC and FISH for *HER2*-overexpressing NSCLC patients has been already utilized in clinical trials with *HER2*-targeted therapies and continues to be an important tool.[357, 392–394]

Despite the shortcomings of IHC, it provides a widely accessible and cost-effective screening option for fusions and a valuable tool for centers that may not have access to upfront molecular testing, since the majority of ALK-, ROS1-, NTRK-, and RET IHC-negative NSCLC would not require further testing.[382]

10.1.2 Fluorescence in situ Hybridization

FISH can be used for detecting gene rearrangements including fusions, gene amplifications, and polysomy. It is considered the standard for detecting *ALK* and *RET* rearrangements given its high sensitivity and ability to detect fusions independent of partner genes while not requiring a large amount of tissue.[374, 395, 396]

However, FISH is more expensive than IHC and requires a more labor-intensive process. FISH interpretation is not routinely employed in every pathology laboratory and therefore may require expertise that is available only in larger centers or specialty laboratories.[374, 395, 396] Moreover, FISH is difficult to automate fully and cannot be multiplexed. When fusion probes are used, both fusion partners must be targeted to see their chromosomal juxtaposition. On the other hand, break apart probes allow for detection without knowledge of the fusion partner and therefore has broader application. However, shorter inversions or intrachromosomal translocations such as occurs with *NTRK1* fusions can be missed.[397]

Although there are many limitations with FISH and although it may not be a front-line testing strategy for less prevalent mutations such as *NTRK* fusions where NGS would be preferred,[317] it is still considered the standard for confirmation in both IHC and as an orthogonal test for multiplex NGS.[398]

10.1.3 Tissue-Based NGS

Multiplex testing for gene mutations has largely replaced individual RT-PCR analysis, since the former provides simultaneous analysis of numerous genes with high sensitivity when applied to samples of limited size. Moreover, rapid advances in technology have reduced turnaround times and made NGS practical for use in real-time clinical applications. NGS has now become a vital diagnostic tool for NSCLC patients and one of the most common techniques for analyzing DNA and/or RNA in either targeted panel or whole genome (WGS) or whole transcriptome (WTS) sequencing. However, given that WGS and WTS both have time lags and added expense, this has limited their routine use to larger high-volume institutions. NGS readily provides detailed mutational data on key drive oncogenes that we have discussed in this Element, including *EGFR, ALK, ROS1, B-RAF, MET, KRAS, RET, NTRK*, and *ERBB2 (HER2)*, along with hundreds to thousands of other genes that may have potential clinical roles.[399] RNA-based transcriptome sequencing has an added advantage of detecting fusions and splicing isoforms without the intervening introns and allow for quantification of fusion transcripts. While both DNA and RNA methods can detect fusions, RNA methods are increasingly in use.[400]

The disadvantages with all tissue-based NGS methods are turnaround time of one to two weeks, higher per sample cost, and need for a larger tumor sample with adequate cellularity compared to IHC and FISH. These limitations must be addressed due to the need to detect activation of an expanding menu of targetable oncogenes. Despite these limitations, tissue-based NGS overall is established as an essential diagnostic tool in NSCLC diagnosis and management.

10.2 Circulating Tumor DNA

10.2.1 Basic Technology

An emerging diagnostic tool that has been gaining importance in clinical oncology and has been used for patients with NSCLC is the "liquid biopsy" of serum for analysis of ctDNA. A liquid biopsy refers to circulating ctDNA. Also, circulating tumor cells and tumor RNA has been analyzed from serum, but, when detected, tumor DNA thus far seems to provide more reproducible results relevant for a larger number of patients. It examines nucleic acids most commonly in processed plasma to test for molecular alterations using targeted PCR assays such as digital-droplet PCR (ddPCR), BEAMing (beads, emulsion, amplification, and magnetics), NGS such as CAPP-Seq, or whole genome/exome sequencing.[401, 402]

10.2.2 Current Applications

The current main applications of liquid biopsies with ctDNA are either as a complementary role to other diagnostic methods, or as the sole diagnostic tool in those who are generally unfit for invasive tissue sampling or there is insufficient material for molecular analysis of oncogenes. They have demonstrated in multiple studies to be reliable in identifying oncogenic biomarkers such as *EGFR, KRAS, MET,* and *B-RAF* mutations and *ALK* and *ROS1* rearrangements but also increase mutation detection rates by as high as 35–48% in metastatic NSCLC patients along with high specificity rates of >95% and concordance rates of up to 80–90% with tissue genotyping.[401, 403–409]

10.2.3 Emerging Uses

An important emerging application of liquid biopsy has been to use ctDNA to detect early progression and analyze resistance mutations to adapt treatment and monitor dynamic changes under treatment pressures.[410–414] A potential diagnostic schema is displayed in Figure 4.

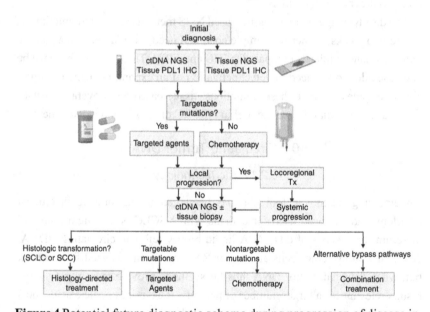

Figure 4 Potential future diagnostic schema during progression of disease in advanced/metastatic NSCLC. A proposed design algorithm that incorporates using upfront ctDNA and whether a repeat biopsy is obtained or not to determine mutation and alterations at the time of resistance. If a biopsy is conducted, then treatment would be based on if there any detectable actionable mutations or a new histologic change and transformation. Figure 4 was created with assistance with biorender.com

[a] Given that there are no guidelines on how to manage bypass alternatives pathways, further research is needed on how to manage these resistance mechanisms and whether combination treatment is able to overcome both the initial oncogene driver and bypass pathways.

Abbreviations: SCC, squamous cell carcinoma; SCLC, small-cell lung cancer; Tx, treatment

Furthermore, ctDNA itself has been evaluated as a possible predictive bio-marker to monitor response to therapy.[415] Previous retrospective studies have shown that patients with *EGFR* and *METex14* mutations that were detected in plasma had similar RRs and outcomes to TKI treatments compared with patients in whom *EGFR* or *METex14* mutations were detected with tissue biopsies.[401, 416–418]

Liquid biopsies still have limited application because, although they have a high specificity, only a minority of patients have detectable ctDNA at diagnosis, and are often those with more advanced disease.[419] ctDNA itself only represents 0.1–10% of the total circulating DNA pool and its detection is dependent on tumor burden and shedding, which is associated with a patient's tumor stage.[415, 420–422] Additionally, there is a lack of established standards for the analytical performance of cell-free tumor DNA or guidelines on the performance characteristics of this type of testing.

As the utility and availability of liquid biopsies has evolved and expanded, it has already proven to be a valuable tool in the diagnoses of cancer and the detection of treatment response and resistance. There are now other studies examining its use in detecting minimal residual disease after surgery [423, 424] or as a prognostic marker, but further trials are needed to further confirm these results. Given the current challenges of low sensitivity rates in liquid biopsies, currently the role of liquid biopsies is mainly as a diagnostic tool.

References

1 Howlader N, Noone AM, Krapcho M et al. (eds.). SEER Cancer Statistics Review, 1975–2017. National Cancer Institute, Bethesda, MD, https://seer cancer.gov/csr/1975_2017/, based on November 2019 SEER data submission, posted to the SEER website, April 2020.

2 Siegel RL, Miller KD, Fuchs HE et al. Cancer statistics, 2022. CA Cancer J Clin 2022; 72 (1): 7–33.

3 Howlader N, Forjaz G, Mooradian MJ et al. The effect of advances in lung-cancer treatment on population mortality. N Engl J Med 2020; 383 (7): 640–649.

4 Palmer RH, Vernersson E, Grabbe C et al. Anaplastic lymphoma kinase: Signalling in development and disease. Biochem J 2009; 420 (3): 345–361.

5 Stoica GE, Kuo A, Aigner A et al. Identification of anaplastic lymphoma kinase as a receptor for the growth factor pleiotrophin. J Biol Chem 2001; 276 (20): 16772–16779.

6 Morris SW, Kirstein MN, Valentine MB et al. Fusion of a kinase gene, ALK, to a nucleolar protein gene, NPM, in non-Hodgkin's lymphoma. Science 1994; 263 (5151): 1281–1284.

7 Murga-Zamalloa C, Lim MS. ALK-driven tumors and targeted therapy: Focus on crizotinib. Pharmgenomics Pers Med 2014; 7: 87–94.

8 Kadomatsu K, Muramatsu T. Midkine and pleiotrophin in neural development and cancer. Cancer Lett 2004; 204 (2): 127–143.

9 Iwahara T, Fujimoto J, Wen D et al. Molecular characterization of ALK, a receptor tyrosine kinase expressed specifically in the nervous system. Oncogene 1997; 14 (4): 439–449.

10 Mossé YP, Wood A, Maris JM. Inhibition of ALK signaling for cancer therapy. Clin Cancer Res 2009; 15 (18): 5609–5614.

11 Rodig SJ, Mino-Kenudson M, Dacic S et al. Unique clinicopathologic features characterize *ALK*-rearranged lung adenocarcinoma in the western population. Clin Cancer Res 2009; 15 (16): 5216–5223.

12 Lou N-N, Zhang X-C, Chen H-J et al. Clinical outcomes of advanced non-small-cell lung cancer patients with EGFR mutation, ALK rearrangement and EGFR/ALK co-alterations. Oncotarget 2016; 7 (40): 65185–65195.

13 Sasaki T, Koivunen J, Ogino A et al. A novel ALK secondary mutation and EGFR signaling cause resistance to ALK kinase inhibitors. Cancer Res 2011; 71 (18): 6051–6060.

14 Soda M, Choi YL, Enomoto M et al. Identification of the transforming EML4-ALK fusion gene in non-small-cell lung cancer. Nature 2007; 448 (7153): 561–566.

15 Rikova K, Guo A, Zeng Q et al. Global survey of phosphotyrosine signaling identifies oncogenic kinases in lung cancer. Cell 2007; 131 (6): 1190–1203.

16 Gristina V, La Mantia M, Iacono F et al. The emerging therapeutic landscape of ALK inhibitors in non-small cell lung cancer. Pharmaceuticals (Basel) 2020; 13 (12): E474.

17 Hallberg B, Palmer RH. Mechanistic insight into ALK receptor tyrosine kinase in human cancer biology. Nat Rev Cancer 2013; 13 (10): 685–700.

18 Takeuchi K, Choi YL, Soda M et al. Multiplex reverse transcription-PCR screening for EML4-ALK fusion transcripts. Clin Cancer Res 2008; 14 (20): 6618–6624.

19 Camidge DR, Dziadziuszko R, Peters S et al. Updated efficacy and safety data and impact of the EML4-ALK fusion variant on the efficacy of alectinib in untreated *ALK*-positive advanced non-small cell lung cancer in the Global Phase III ALEX Study. J Thorac Oncol 2019; 14 (7): 1233–1243.

20 Christensen JG, Zou HY, Arango ME et al. Cytoreductive antitumor activity of PF-2341066, a novel inhibitor of anaplastic lymphoma kinase and c-Met, in experimental models of anaplastic large-cell lymphoma. Mol Cancer Ther 2007; 6 (12 pt. 1): 3314–3322.

21 Kwak EL, Bang Y-J, Camidge DR et al. Anaplastic lymphoma kinase inhibition in non-small-cell lung cancer. N Engl J Med 2010; 363 (18): 1693–1703.

22 Blackhall F, Ross Camidge D, Shaw AT et al. Final results of the large-scale multinational trial PROFILE 1005: Efficacy and safety of crizotinib in previously treated patients with advanced/metastatic *ALK*-positive non-small-cell lung cancer. ESMO Open 2017; 2 (3): e000219.

23 Shaw AT, Kim D-W, Nakagawa K et al. Crizotinib versus chemotherapy in advanced *ALK*-positive lung cancer. N Engl J Med 2013; 368 (25): 2385–2394.

24 Solomon BJ, Mok T, Kim D-W et al. First-line crizotinib versus chemotherapy in *ALK*-positive lung cancer. N Engl J Med 2014; 371 (23): 2167–2177.

25 Kim D-W, Mehra R, Tan DSW et al. Activity and safety of ceritinib in patients with *ALK*-rearranged non-small-cell lung cancer (ASCEND-1): Updated results from the multicentre, open-label, phase 1 trial. Lancet Oncol 2016; 17 (4): 452–463.

26 Crinò L, Ahn M-J, De Marinis F et al. Multicenter phase II study of whole-body and intracranial activity with ceritinib in patients with

ALK-rearranged non-small-cell lung cancer previously treated with chemotherapy and crizotinib: Results from ASCEND-2. J Clin Oncol 2016; 34 (24): 2866–2873.

27 Soria J-C, Tan DSW, Chiari R et al. First-line ceritinib versus platinum-based chemotherapy in advanced *ALK*-rearranged non-small-cell lung cancer (ASCEND-4): A randomised, open-label, phase 3 study. Lancet 2017; 389 (10072): 917–929.

28 Shaw AT, Kim TM, Crinò L et al. Ceritinib versus chemotherapy in patients with *ALK*-rearranged non-small-cell lung cancer previously given chemotherapy and crizotinib (ASCEND-5): A randomised, controlled, open-label, phase 3 trial. Lancet Oncol 2017; 18 (7): 874–886.

29 Seto T, Kiura K, Nishio M et al. CH5424802 (RO5424802) for patients with *ALK*-rearranged advanced non-small-cell lung cancer (AF-001JP study): A single-arm, open-label, phase 1–2 study. Lancet Oncol 2013; 14 (7): 590–598.

30 Shaw AT, Gandhi L, Gadgeel S et al. Alectinib in *ALK*-positive, crizotinib-resistant, non-small-cell lung cancer: A single-group, multicentre, phase 2 trial. Lancet Oncol 2016; 17 (2): 234–242.

31 Nakagawa K, Hida T, Nokihara H et al. Final progression-free survival results from the J-ALEX study of alectinib versus crizotinib in *ALK*-positive non-small-cell lung cancer. Lung Cancer 2020; 139: 195–199.

32 Yoshioka H, Hida T, Nokihara H et al. Final OS analysis from the phase III J-ALEX study of alectinib (ALC) versus crizotinib (CRZ) in Japanese ALK-inhibitor naïve *ALK*-positive non-small cell lung cancer (ALK+ NSCLC). J Clin Oncol 2021; 39 (15 suppl.): 9022.

33 Peters S, Camidge DR, Shaw AT et al. Alectinib versus crizotinib in untreated *ALK*-positive non-small-cell lung cancer. N Engl J Med 2017; 377 (9): 829–838.

34 Mok T, Camidge DR, Gadgeel SM et al. Updated overall survival and final progression-free survival data for patients with treatment-naive advanced *ALK*-positive non-small-cell lung cancer in the ALEX study. Ann Oncol 2020; 31 (8): 1056–1064.

35 Gadgeel S, Peters S, Mok T et al. Alectinib versus crizotinib in treatment-naive anaplastic lymphoma kinase-positive (ALK+) non-small-cell lung cancer: CNS efficacy results from the ALEX study. Ann Oncol 2018; 29 (11): 2214–2222.

36 Kim DW, Tiseo M, Ahn MJ et al. Brigatinib in patients with crizotinib-refractory anaplastic lymphoma kinase-positive non-small-cell lung cancer: A randomized, multicenter phase II trial. J Clin Oncol 2017; 35 (22): 2490–2498.

37 Huber RM, Hansen KH, Paz-Ares Rodríguez L et al. Brigatinib in crizotinib-refractory ALK+ NSCLC: 2-year follow-up on systemic and intra-cranial outcomes in the phase 2 ALTA trial. J Thorac Oncol 2020; 15 (3): 404–415.

38 Camidge DR, Kim HR, Ahn M-J et al. Brigatinib versus crizotinib in *ALK*-positive non-small-cell lung cancer. N Engl J Med 2018; 379 (21): 2027–2039.

39 Camidge DR, Kim HR, Ahn M-J et al. Brigatinib versus crizotinib in advanced ALK inhibitor-naive *ALK*-positive non-small cell lung cancer: Second interim analysis of the phase III ALTA-1L trial. J Clin Oncol 2020; 38 (31): 3592–3603.

40 Solomon BJ, Besse B, Bauer TM et al. Lorlatinib in patients with *ALK*-positive non-small-cell lung cancer: Results from a global phase 2 study. Lancet Oncol 2018; 19 (12): 1654–1667.

41 Shaw AT, Bauer TM, de Marinis F et al. First-line lorlatinib or crizotinib in advanced *ALK*-positive lung cancer.N Engl J Med 2020; 383 (21): 2018–2029.

42 Gainor JF, Shaw AT. Emerging paradigms in the development of resistance to tyrosine kinase inhibitors in lung cancer. J Clin Oncol 2013; 31 (31): 3987–3996.

43 Gainor JF, Dardaei L, Yoda S et al. Molecular mechanisms of resistance to first- and second-generation ALK inhibitors in *ALK*-rearranged lung cancer. Cancer Discov 2016; 6 (10): 1118–1133.

44 Lin JJ, Zhu VW, Yoda S et al. Impact of EML4-ALK variant on resistance mechanisms and clinical outcomes in *ALK*-positive lung cancer. J Clin Oncol 2018; 36 (12): 1199–1206.

45 Lucena-Araujo AR, Moran JP, VanderLaan PA et al. De novo ALK kinase domain mutations are uncommon in kinase inhibitor-naïve *ALK* rearranged lung cancers. Lung Cancer 2016; 99: 17–22.

46 Shaw AT, Felip E, Bauer TM et al. Lorlatinib in non-small-cell lung cancer with ALK or ROS1 rearrangement: An international, multicentre, open-label, single-arm first-in-man phase 1 trial. Lancet Oncol 2017; 18 (12): 1590–1599.

47 Shaw AT, Solomon BJ, Besse B et al. ALK resistance mutations and efficacy of lorlatinib in advanced anaplastic lymphoma kinase-positive non-small-cell lung cancer. J Clin Oncol 2019; 37 (16): 1370–1379.

48 Smolle E, Taucher V, Lindenmann J et al. Current knowledge about mechanisms of drug resistance against ALK inhibitors in non-small cell lung cancer. Cancers (Basel) 2021; 13 (4): 699.

49 Tyner JW, Fletcher LB, Wang EQ et al. MET receptor sequence variants R970C and T992I lack transforming capacity. Cancer Res 2010; 70 (15): 6233–6237.

50 Guarino M, Rubino B, Ballabio G. The role of epithelial-mesenchymal transition in cancer pathology. Pathology 2007; 39 (3): 305–318.

51 Fukuda K, Takeuchi S, Arai S et al. Epithelial-to-mesenchymal transition is a mechanism of ALK inhibitor resistance in lung cancer independent of ALK mutation status. Cancer Res 2019; 79 (7): 1658–1670.

52 Cha YJ, Cho BC, Kim HR et al. A case of *ALK*-rearranged adenocarcinoma with small cell carcinoma-like transformation and resistance to crizotinib. J Thorac Oncol 2016; 11 (5): e55–e58.

53 D'Incecco A, Andreozzi M, Ludovini V et al. PD-1 and PD-L1 expression in molecularly selected non-small-cell lung cancer patients. Br J Cancer 2015; 112 (1): 95–102.

54 Hong S, Chen N, Fang W et al. Upregulation of PD-L1 by EML4-ALK fusion protein mediates the immune escape in ALK positive NSCLC: Implication for optional anti-PD-1/PD-L1 immune therapy for ALK-TKIs sensitive and resistant NSCLC patients. Oncoimmunology 2016; 5 (3): e1094598.

55 Gainor JF, Shaw AT, Sequist LV et al. EGFR mutations and ALK rearrangements are associated with low response rates to PD-1 pathway blockade in non-small cell lung cancer: A retrospective analysis. Clin Cancer Res 2016; 22 (18): 4585–4593.

56 Spigel DR, Reynolds C, Waterhouse D et al. Phase 1/2 study of the safety and tolerability of nivolumab plus crizotinib for the first-line treatment of anaplastic lymphoma kinase translocation-positive advanced non-small cell lung cancer (CheckMate 370). J Thorac Oncol 2018; 13 (5): 682–688.

57 Sakamoto H, Tsukaguchi T, Hiroshima S et al. CH5424802, a selective ALK inhibitor capable of blocking the resistant gatekeeper mutant. Cancer Cell 2011; 19 (5): 679–690.

58 Solomon BJ, Ahn JS, Barlesi F et al. ALINA: A phase III study of alectinib versus chemotherapy as adjuvant therapy in patients with stage IB–IIIA anaplastic lymphoma kinase-positive (ALK+) non-small cell lung cancer (NSCLC). J Clin Oncol 2019; 37 (15 suppl.): TPS8569.

59 Horn L, Wang Z, Wu G et al. Ensartinib vs crizotinib for patients with anaplastic lymphoma kinase-positive non-small cell lung cancer: A randomized clinical trial. JAMA Oncol 2021; 7 (11): 1617–1625.

60 Yang J-J, Zhou J, Yang N et al. SAF-189s in previously treated patients with advanced *ALK*-rearranged non-small cell lung cancer (NSCLC): Results from the dose-finding portion in a single-arm, first-in-human phase I/II study. J Clin Oncol 2020; 38 (15 suppl.): e21689.

61 Fang Y, Pan H, Lu S et al. A phase I study to evaluate safety, tolerability, pharmacokinetics, and preliminary antitumor activity of TQ-B3101. J Clin Oncol 2020; 38 (15 suppl.): e21705.

62 Murray BW, Zhai D, Deng W et al. TPX-0131, a potent CNS-penetrant, next-generation inhibitor of wild-type ALK and ALK-resistant mutations. Mol Cancer Ther 2021; 20 (9): 1499–1507.

63 Pelish HE, Tangpeerachaikul A, Kohl NE et al. Abstract 1468: NUV-655 (NVL-655) is a selective, brain-penetrant ALK inhibitor with antitumor activity against the lorlatinib-resistant G1202R/L1196M compound mutation. Cancer Res 2021; 81 (13 suppl.): 1468.

64 Uguen A, de Braekeleer M. ROS1 fusions in cancer: A review. Future Oncol 2016; 12 (16): 1911–1928.

65 Acquaviva J, Wong R, Charest A. The multifaceted roles of the receptor tyrosine kinase ROS in development and cancer. Biochim Biophys Acta 2009; 1795 (1): 37–52.

66 Birchmeier C, Sharma S, Wigler M. Expression and rearrangement of the *ROS1* gene in human glioblastoma cells. Proc Natl Acad Sci USA 1987; 84 (24): 9270–9274.

67 Gu T-L, Deng X, Huang F et al. Survey of tyrosine kinase signaling reveals ROS kinase fusions in human cholangiocarcinoma. PLoS One 2011; 6 (1): e15640.

68 Lee J, Lee SE, Kang SY et al. Identification of ROS1 rearrangement in gastric adenocarcinoma. Cancer 2013; 119 (9): 1627–1635.

69 Birch AH, Arcand SL, Oros KK et al. Chromosome 3 anomalies investigated by genome wide SNP analysis of benign, low malignant potential and low grade ovarian serous tumours. PLoS One 2011; 6 (12): e28250.

70 Gainor JF, Shaw AT. Novel targets in non-small cell lung cancer: ROS1 and RET fusions. Oncologist 2013; 18 (7): 865–875.

71 Shaw AT, Riely GJ, Bang YJ et al. Crizotinib in *ROS1*-rearranged advanced non-small-cell lung cancer (NSCLC): Updated results, including overall survival, from PROFILE 1001. Ann Oncol 2019; 30 (7): 1121–1126.

72 Wu Y-L, Yang JC-H, Kim D-W et al. Phase II study of crizotinib in East Asian patients with ROS1-Positive advanced non-small-cell lung cancer. J Clin Oncol 2018; 36 (14): 1405–1411.

73 Michels S, Massutí B, Schildhaus H-U et al. Safety and efficacy of crizotinib in patients with advanced or metastatic *ROS1*-rearranged lung cancer (EUCROSS): A European phase II clinical trial. J Thorac Oncol 2019; 14 (7): 1266–1276.

74 Roys A, Chang X, Liu Y et al. Resistance mechanisms and potent-targeted therapies of *ROS1*-positive lung cancer. Cancer Chemother Pharmacol 2019; 84 (4): 679–688.

75 Lim SM, Kim HR, Lee J-S et al. Open-label, multicenter, phase II study of ceritinib in patients with non-small-cell lung cancer harboring ROS1 rearrangement. J Clin Oncol 2017; 35 (23): 2613–2618.

76 Azelby CM, Sakamoto MR, Bowles DW. ROS1 targeted therapies: Current status. Curr Oncol Rep 2021; 23 (8): 94.

77 Ardini E, Menichincheri M, Banfi P et al. Entrectinib, a pan-TRK, ROS1, and ALK inhibitor with activity in multiple molecularly defined cancer indications. Mol Cancer Ther 2016; 15 (4): 628–639.

78 Drilon A, Siena S, Dziadziuszko R et al. Entrectinib in ROS1 fusion-positive non-small-cell lung cancer: Integrated analysis of three phase 1–2 trials. Lancet Oncol 2020; 21 (2): 261–270.

79 Barlesi F, Drilon A, Braud FD et al. Entrectinib in locally advanced or metastatic ROS1 fusion-positive non-small cell lung cancer (NSCLC): Integrated analysis of ALKA-372–001, STARTRK-1 and STARTRK-2. Ann Oncol 2019; 30: ii48–ii49.

80 Shaw AT, Solomon BJ, Chiari R et al. Lorlatinib in advanced ROS1-positive non-small-cell lung cancer: A multicentre, open-label, single-arm, phase 1–2 trial. Lancet Oncol 2019; 20 (12): 1691–1701.

81 Lin JJ, Choudhury NJ, Yoda S et al. Spectrum of mechanisms of resistance to crizotinib and lorlatinib in ROS1 fusion-positive lung cancer. Clin Cancer Res 2021; 27 (10): 2899–2909.

82 Drilon A, Somwar R, Wagner JP et al. A novel crizotinib-resistant solvent-front mutation responsive to cabozantinib therapy in a patient with *ROS1*-rearranged lung cancer. Clin Cancer Res 2016; 22 (10): 2351–2358.

83 Drilon A, Ou S-HI, Cho BC et al. Repotrectinib (TPX-0005) Is a next-generation ROS1/TRK/ALK inhibitor that potently inhibits ROS1/ TRK/ALK solvent-front mutations. Cancer Discov 2018; 8 (10): 1227–1236.

84 Cho BC, Doebele RC, Lin J et al. MA11.07 phase 1/2 TRIDENT-1 study of repotrectinib in patients with ROS1+ or NTRK+ advanced solid tumors. J Thorac Oncol 2021; 16 (3): S174–S175.

85 Ou SI, Fujiwara Y, Shaw AT et al. Efficacy of taletrectinib (AB-106/DS-6051b) in ROS1+ NSCLC: An updated pooled analysis of U.S. and Japan phase 1 studies. JTO Clin Res Rep 2021; 2 (1): 100108.

86 Zhou C, Fan H, Wang Y et al. Taletrectinib (AB-106; DS-6051b) in metastatic non-small cell lung cancer (NSCLC) patients with ROS1 fusion: Preliminary results of TRUST. J Clin Oncol 2021; 39 (15 suppl.): 9066.

87 Ai X, Wang Q, Cheng Y et al. Safety but limited efficacy of ensartinib in *ROS1*-positive NSCLC: A single-arm, multicenter phase 2 study. J Thorac Oncol 2021; 16 (11): 1959–1963.

88 Takahashi M, Ritz J, Cooper GM. Activation of a novel human transforming gene, ret, by DNA rearrangement. Cell 1985; 42 (2): 581–588.

89 Ibanez CF. Structure and physiology of the RET receptor tyrosine kinase. Cold Spring Harb Perspect Biol 2013; 5 (2).

90 Besset V, Scott RP, Ibanez CF. Signaling complexes and protein-protein interactions involved in the activation of the Ras and phosphatidylinositol 3-kinase pathways by the c-Ret receptor tyrosine kinase. J Biol Chem 2000; 275 (50): 39159–39166.

91 Coulpier M, Anders J, Ibanez CF. Coordinated activation of autophosphorylation sites in the RET receptor tyrosine kinase: Importance of tyrosine 1062 for GDNF mediated neuronal differentiation and survival. J Biol Chem 2002; 277 (3): 1991–1999.

92 De Vita G, Melillo RM, Carlomagno F et al. Tyrosine 1062 of RET-MEN2A mediates activation of Akt (protein kinase B) and mitogen-activated protein kinase pathways leading to PC12 cell survival. Cancer Res 2000; 60 (14): 3727–3731.

93 Jain S, Encinas M, Johnson EM, Jr. et al. Critical and distinct roles for key RET tyrosine docking sites in renal development. Genes Dev 2006; 20 (3): 321–333.

94 Jijiwa M, Kawai K, Fukihara J et al. GDNF-mediated signaling via RET tyrosine 1062 is essential for maintenance of spermatogonial stem cells. Genes Cells 2008; 13 (4): 365–374.

95 Romei C, Ciampi R, Elisei R. A comprehensive overview of the role of the RET proto-oncogene in thyroid carcinoma. Nat Rev Endocrinol 2016; 12 (4): 192–202.

96 Santoro M, Moccia M, Federico G et al. RET gene fusions in malignancies of the thyroid and other tissues. Genes (Basel) 2020; 11 (4).

97 Larouche V, Akirov A, Thomas CM et al. A primer on the genetics of medullary thyroid cancer. Curr Oncol 2019; 26 (6): 389–394.

98 Fagin JA, Wells SA, Jr. Biologic and clinical perspectives on thyroid cancer. N Engl J Med 2016; 375 (11): 1054–1067.

99 Grubbs EG, Ng PK, Bui J et al. RET fusion as a novel driver of medullary thyroid carcinoma. J Clin Endocrinol Metab 2015; 100 (3): 788–793.

100 Kohno T, Tabata J, Nakaoku T. REToma: A cancer subtype with a shared driver oncogene. Carcinogenesis 2020; 41 (2): 123–129.

101 Yakushina VD, Lerner LV, Lavrov AV. Gene fusions in thyroid cancer. Thyroid 2018; 28 (2): 158–167.

102 Accardo G, Conzo G, Esposito D et al. Genetics of medullary thyroid cancer: An overview. Int J Surg 2017; 41 (suppl. 1): S2–S6.

103 Li AY, McCusker MG, Russo A et al. RET fusions in solid tumors. Cancer Treat Rev 2019; 81: 101911.

104 Drilon A, Lin JJ, Filleron T et al. Frequency of brain metastases and multikinase inhibitor outcomes in patients with *RET*-rearranged lung cancers. J Thorac Oncol 2018; 13 (10): 1595–1601.

105 Gautschi O, Milia J, Filleron T et al. Targeting RET in patients with *RET*-rearranged lung cancers: Results From the global, multicenter RET registry. J Clin Oncol 2017; 35 (13): 1403–1410.

106 Drilon A, Hu ZI, Lai GGY et al. Targeting RET-driven cancers: Lessons from evolving preclinical and clinical landscapes. Nat Rev Clin Oncol 2018; 15 (3): 151–167.

107 Hess LM, Han Y, Zhu YE et al. Characteristics and outcomes of patients with RET-fusion positive non-small lung cancer in real-world practice in the United States. BMC Cancer 2021; 21 (1): 28.

108 Drilon A, Oxnard GR, Tan DSW et al. Efficacy of selpercatinib in RET fusion-positive non-small-cell lung cancer. N Engl J Med 2020; 383 (9): 813–824.

109 Kato S, Subbiah V, Marchlik E et al. RET aberrations in diverse cancers: Next-generation sequencing of 4,871 patients. Clin Cancer Res 2017; 23 (8): 1988–1997.

110 Morra F, Luise C, Visconti R et al. New therapeutic perspectives in CCDC6 deficient lung cancer cells. Int J Cancer 2015; 136 (9): 2146–2157.

111 Bellelli R, Castellone MD, Guida T et al. NCOA4 transcriptional coactivator inhibits activation of DNA replication origins. Mol Cell 2014; 55 (1): 123–137.

112 Das TK, Cagan RL. KIF5B-RET oncoprotein signals through a multi-kinase signaling hub. Cell Rep 2017; 20 (10): 2368–2383.

113 Vaishnavi A, Schubert L, Rix U et al. EGFR mediates responses to small-molecule drugs targeting oncogenic fusion kinases. Cancer Res 2017; 77 (13): 3551–3563.

114 Nakaoku T, Kohno T, Araki M et al. A secondary RET mutation in the activation loop conferring resistance to vandetanib. Nat Commun 2018; 9 (1): 625.

115 Hida T, Velcheti V, Reckamp KL et al. A phase 2 study of lenvatinib in patients with RET fusion-positive lung adenocarcinoma. Lung Cancer 2019; 138: 124–130.

116 Drilon A, Rekhtman N, Arcila M et al. Cabozantinib in patients with advanced *RET*-rearranged non-small-cell lung cancer: An open-label, single-centre, phase 2, single-arm trial. Lancet Oncol 2016; 17 (12): 1653–1660.

117 Drilon A, Wang L, Hasanovic A et al. Response to cabozantinib in patients with RET fusion-positive lung adenocarcinomas. Cancer Discov 2013; 3 (6): 630–635.

118 Lee SH, Lee JK, Ahn MJ et al. Vandetanib in pretreated patients with advanced non-small cell lung cancer-harboring RET rearrangement: A phase II clinical trial. Ann Oncol 2017; 28 (2): 292–297.

119 Hayman SR, Leung N, Grande JP et al. VEGF inhibition, hypertension, and renal toxicity. Curr Oncol Rep 2012; 14 (4): 285–294.

120 Lacouture ME, Anadkat MJ, Bensadoun RJ et al. Clinical practice guidelines for the prevention and treatment of EGFR inhibitor-associated dermatologic toxicities. Support Care Cancer 2011; 19 (8): 1079–1095.

121 Choudhury NJ, Drilon A. Decade in review: A new era for *RET*-rearranged lung cancers. Transl Lung Cancer Res 2020; 9 (6): 2571–2580.

122 Fancelli S, Caliman E, Mazzoni F et al. Chasing the target: New phenomena of resistance to novel selective RET inhibitors in lung cancer. Updated evidence and future perspectives. Cancers (Basel) 2021; 13 (5).

123 Gainor JF, Curigliano G, Kim D-W et al. Pralsetinib for RET fusion-positive non-small-cell lung cancer (ARROW): A multi-cohort, open-label, phase 1/2 study.Lancet Oncol 2021; 22 (7): 959–969.

124 Chang H, Sung JH, Moon SU et al. EGF induced RET inhibitor resistance in CCDC6-RET lung cancer cells. Yonsei Med J 2017; 58 (1): 9–18.

125 Blakely CM, Watkins TBK, Wu W et al. Evolution and clinical impact of co-occurring genetic alterations in advanced-stage EGFR-mutant lung cancers. Nat Genet 2017; 49 (12): 1693–1704.

126 Suda K, Mitsudomi T. Emerging oncogenic fusions other than ALK, ROS1, RET, and NTRK in NSCLC and the role of fusions as resistance mechanisms to targeted therapy. Transl Lung Cancer Res 2020; 9 (6): 2618–2628.

127 Piotrowska Z, Isozaki H, Lennerz JK et al. Landscape of acquired resistance to osimertinib in EGFR-mutant NSCLC and clinical validation of combined EGFR and RET inhibition with osimertinib and BLU-667 for acquired RET fusion. Cancer Discov 2018; 8 (12): 1529–1539.

128 Rich TA, Reckamp KL, Chae YK et al. Analysis of cell-free DNA from 32,989 advanced cancers reveals novel co-occurring activating RET alterations and oncogenic signaling pathway aberrations. Clin Cancer Res 2019; 25 (19): 5832–5842.

129 Rotow J, Patel J, Hanley M et al. FP14.07 combination osimertinib plus selpercatinib for EGFR-mutant non-small cell lung cancer (NSCLC) with acquired RET fusions. J Thorac Oncol 2021; 16 (3).

130 Turning Point Therapeutics. Turning Point Therapeutics Announces Initial Clinical Data from Phase 1/2 SWORD-1 Study of RET Inhibitor TPX-0046. Turning Point Therapeutics, San Diego, CA, April 7, 2021.

131 Schoffski P, Cho BC, Italiano A et al. BOS172738, a highly potent and selective RET inhibitor, for the treatment of *RET*-altered tumors including RET-fusion+ NSCLC and RET-mutant MTC: Phase 1 study results. J Clin Oncol 2021; 39 (15 suppl.): 3008.

132 Moccia M, Frett B, Zhang L et al. Bioisosteric discovery of NPA101.3, a second-generation RET/VEGFR2 inhibitor optimized for single-agent polypharmacology. J Med Chem 2020; 63 (9): 4506–4516.

133 Cooper CS PM, Blair DG, Tainsky MA et al. Molecular cloning of a new transforming gene from a chemically transformed human cell line. Nature 1984; 311 (5981): 29–33.

134 Furge KA, Zhang YW, Vande Woude GF. Met receptor tyrosine kinase: Enhanced signaling through adapter proteins. Oncogene 2000; 19 (49): 5582–5589.

135 Skead G, Govender D. Gene of the month: *MET.* J Clin Pathol 2015; 68 (6): 405–409.

136 Birchmeier C, Birchmeier W, Gherardi E et al. Met, metastasis, motility and more. Nat Rev Mol Cell Biol 2003; 4 (12): 915–925.

137 Cecchi F, Rabe DC, Bottaro DP. Targeting the HGF/Met signaling pathway in cancer therapy. Expert Opin Ther Targets 2012; 16 (6): 553–572.

138 Kolatsi-Joannou M, Moore R, Winyard PJ et al. Expression of hepatocyte growth factor/scatter factor and its receptor, MET, suggests roles in human embryonic organogenesis. Pediatr Res 1997; 41 (5): 657–665.

139 Reungwetwattana T, Liang Y, Zhu V et al. The race to target *MET exon 14* skipping alterations in non-small cell lung cancer: The why, the how, the who, the unknown, and the inevitable. Lung Cancer 2017; 103: 27–37.

140 Lamberti G, Andrini E, Sisi M et al. Beyond EGFR, ALK and ROS1: Current evidence and future perspectives on newly targetable oncogenic drivers in lung adenocarcinoma. Crit Rev Oncol Hematol 2020; 156: 103119.

141 Deheuninck J, Goormachtigh G, Foveau B et al. Phosphorylation of the MET receptor on juxtamembrane tyrosine residue 1001 inhibits its caspase-dependent cleavage. Cell Signal 2009; 21 (9): 1455–1463.

142 Peschard P, Fournier TM, Lamorte L et al. Mutation of the c-Cbl TKB domain binding site on the MET receptor tyrosine kinase converts it into a transforming protein. Molecular Cell 2001; 8 (5): 995–1004.

143 Cortot AB, Kherrouche Z, Descarpentries C et al. Exon 14 deleted MET receptor as a new biomarker and target in cancers. J Natl Cancer Inst 2017; 109 (5).

144 Cheng TL, Chang MY, Huang SY et al. Overexpression of circulating c-met messenger RNA is significantly correlated with nodal stage and early recurrence in non-small cell lung cancer. Chest 2005; 128 (3): 1453–1460.

145 Ma PC, Jagadeeswaran R, Jagadeesh S et al. Functional expression and mutations of c-Met and its therapeutic inhibition with SU11274 and small interfering RNA in non-small cell lung cancer. Cancer Res 2005; 65 (4): 1479–1488.

146 Socinski MA, Pennell NA, Davies KD. *MET exon 14* skipping mutations in non-small-cell lung cancer: An overview of biology, clinical outcomes, and testing considerations. JCO Precis Oncol 2021; 5.

147 Schrock AB, Frampton GM, Suh J et al. Characterization of 298 patients with lung cancer harboring *MET exon 14* skipping alterations. J Thorac Oncol 2016; 11 (9): 1493–1502.

148 Liu X, Jia Y, Stoopler MB et al. Next-generation sequencing of pulmonary sarcomatoid carcinoma reveals high frequency of actionable *MET* gene mutations. J Clin Oncol 2016; 34 (8): 794–802.

149 Awad MM, Oxnard GR, Jackman DM et al. *MET exon 14* mutations in non-small-cell lung cancer are associated with advanced age and stage-dependent MET genomic amplification and c-MET overexpression. J Clin Oncol 2016; 34 (7): 721–730.

150 Digumarthy SR, Mendoza DP, Zhang EW et al. Clinicopathologic and imaging features of non-small-cell lung cancer with *MET exon 14* skipping mutations. Cancers (Basel) 2019; 11 (12).

151 Lee GD, Lee SE, Oh DY et al. *MET exon 14* skipping mutations in lung adenocarcinoma: Clinicopathologic implications and prognostic values. J Thorac Oncol 2017; 12 (8): 1233–1246.

152 Tong JH, Yeung SF, Chan AW et al. MET amplification and exon 14 splice site mutation define unique molecular subgroups of non-small cell lung carcinoma with poor prognosis. Clin Cancer Res 2016; 22 (12): 3048–3056.

153 Awad MM, Leonardi GC, Kravets S et al. Impact of MET inhibitors on survival among patients with non-small cell lung cancer harboring *MET exon 14* mutations: A retrospective analysis. Lung Cancer 2019; 133: 96–102.

154 Awad MM, Lee JK, Madison R et al. Characterization of 1,387 NSCLCs with *MET exon 14* (*METex14*) skipping alterations (SA) and potential acquired resistance (AR) mechanisms. J Clin Oncol 2020; 38 (15 suppl.): 9511.

155 Frampton GM, Ali SM, Rosenzweig M et al. Activation of MET via diverse exon 14 splicing alterations occurs in multiple tumor types and

confers clinical sensitivity to MET inhibitors. Cancer Discov 2015; 5 (8): 850–859.

156 Lee JK, Madison R, Classon A et al. Characterization of non-small-cell lung cancers with *MET exon 14* skipping alterations detected in tissue or liquid: Clinicogenomics and real-world treatment patterns. JCO Precis Oncol 2021; 5.

157 Drilon A, Clark JW, Weiss J et al. Antitumor activity of crizotinib in lung cancers harboring a *MET exon 14* alteration. Nat Med 2020; 26 (1): 47–51.

158 Landi L, Chiari R, Tiseo M et al. Crizotinib in MET-deregulated or *ROS1*-rearranged pretreated non-small cell lung cancer (METROS): A phase II, prospective, multicenter, two-arms trial. Clin Cancer Res 2019; 25 (24): 7312–7319.

159 Wolf J, Seto T, Han JY et al. Capmatinib in *MET exon 14*-mutated or MET-amplified non-small-cell lung cancer. N Engl J Med 2020; 383 (10): 944–957.

160 Paik PK, Felip E, Veillon R et al. Tepotinib in non-small-cell lung cancer with *MET exon 14* skipping mutations. N Engl J Med 2020; 383 (10): 931–943.

161 Lu S, Fang J, Li X et al. Phase II study of savolitinib in patients (pts) with pulmonary sarcomatoid carcinoma (PSC) and other types of non-small cell lung cancer (NSCLC) harboring *MET exon 14* skipping mutations (METex14+). J Clin Oncol 2020; 38 (15 suppl.): 9519.

162 Wang SXY, Zhang BM, Wakelee HA et al. Case series of *MET exon 14* skipping mutation-positive non-small-cell lung cancers with response to crizotinib and cabozantinib. Anticancer Drugs 2019; 30 (5): 537–541.

163 D'Arcangelo M, Tassinari D, De Marinis F et al. P2.01–15 phase II single arm study of cabozantinib in non-small cell lung cancer patients with MET deregulation (CABinMET). J Thorac Oncol 2019; 14 (10).

164 Suzawa K, Offin M, Schoenfeld AJ et al. Acquired *MET exon 14* alteration drives secondary resistance to epidermal growth factor receptor tyrosine kinase inhibitor in EGFR-mutated lung cancer. JCO Precis Oncol 2019; 3.

165 Heist RS, Sequist LV, Borger D et al. Acquired resistance to crizotinib in NSCLC with *MET exon 14* skipping. J Thorac Oncol 2016; 11 (8): 1242–1245.

166 Recondo G, Bahcall M, Spurr LF et al. Molecular mechanisms of acquired resistance to MET tyrosine kinase inhibitors in patients with *MET exon 14*-mutant NSCLC. Clin Cancer Res 2020; 26 (11): 2615–2625.

167 Bahcall M, Sim T, Paweletz CP et al. Acquired METD1228V mutation and resistance to MET inhibition in lung cancer. Cancer Discov 2016; 6 (12): 1334–1341.

168 Fujino T, Kobayashi Y, Suda K et al. Sensitivity and resistance of *MET exon 14* mutations in lung cancer to eight MET tyrosine kinase inhibitors in vitro. J Thorac Oncol 2019; 14 (10): 1753–1765.

169 Engstrom LD, Aranda R, Lee M et al. Glesatinib exhibits antitumor activity in lung cancer models and patients harboring *MET exon 14* mutations and overcomes mutation-mediated resistance to type I MET inhibitors in nonclinical models. Clin Cancer Res 2017; 23 (21): 6661–6672.

170 Schoenfeld AJ, Chan JM, Kubota D et al. Tumor analyses reveal squamous transformation and off-target alterations as early resistance mechanisms to first-line osimertinib in EGFR-mutant lung cancer. Clin Cancer Res 2020; 26 (11): 2654–2663.

171 Bahcall M, Awad MM, Sholl LM et al. Amplification of wild-type KRAS imparts resistance to crizotinib in *MET exon 14* mutant non-small cell lung cancer. Clin Cancer Res 2018; 24 (23): 5963–5976.

172 Ali SM, Sanford EM, Klempner SJ et al. Prospective comprehensive genomic profiling of advanced gastric carcinoma cases reveals frequent clinically relevant genomic alterations and new routes for targeted therapies. Oncologist 2015; 20 (5): 499–507.

173 Bardelli A, Corso S, Bertotti A et al. Amplification of the MET receptor drives resistance to anti-EGFR therapies in colorectal cancer. Cancer Discov 2013; 3 (6): 658–673.

174 Okuda K, Sasaki H, Yukiue H et al. Met gene copy number predicts the prognosis for completely resected non-small cell lung cancer. Cancer Sci 2008; 99 (11): 2280–2285.

175 Kim JH, Kim HS, Kim BJ. Prognostic value of MET copy number gain in non-small-cell lung cancer: An updated meta-analysis. J Cancer 2018; 9 (10): 1836–1845.

176 Noonan SA, Berry L, Lu X et al. Identifying the appropriate FISH criteria for defining MET copy number-driven lung adenocarcinoma through oncogene overlap analysis. J Thorac Oncol 2016; 11 (8): 1293–1304.

177 Camidge DR, Otterson GA, Clark JW et al. Crizotinib in patients (pts) with MET-amplified non-small cell lung cancer (NSCLC): Updated safety and efficacy findings from a phase 1 trial. J Clin Oncol 2018; 36 (15 suppl.): 9062.

178 Ko B, He T, Gadgeel S et al. MET/HGF pathway activation as a paradigm of resistance to targeted therapies. Ann Transl Med 2017; 5 (1): 4.

179 Papadimitrakopoulou VA, Wu YL, Han JY et al. Analysis of resistance mechanisms to osimertinib in patients with EGFR T790M advanced NSCLC from the AURA3 study. Ann Oncol 2018; 29 (52): 20932–20937.

180 Bean J, Brennan C, Shih JY et al. MET amplification occurs with or without T790M mutations in EGFR mutant lung tumors with acquired resistance to gefitinib or erlotinib. Proc Natl Acad Sci USA 2007; 104 (52): 20932–20937.

181 Wu YL, Zhang L, Kim DW et al. Phase Ib/II study of capmatinib (INC280) plus gefitinib after failure of epidermal growth factor receptor (EGFR) inhibitor therapy in patients with EGFR-mutated, MET factor-dysregulated non-small-cell lung cancer. J Clin Oncol 2018; 36 (31): 3101–3109.

182 Wu Y-L, Cheng Y, Zhou J et al. Tepotinib plus gefitinib in patients with EGFR-mutant non-small-cell lung cancer with MET overexpression or MET amplification and acquired resistance to previous EGFR inhibitor (INSIGHT study): An open-label, phase 1b/2, multicentre, randomised trial. Lancet Resp Med 2020; 8 (11): 1132–1143.

183 Deng W, Zhai D, Rogers E et al. Abstract 1325: TPX-0022, a polypharmacology inhibitor of MET/CSF1R/SRC inhibits tumor growth by promoting anti-tumor immune responses. Cancer Res 2019; 79 (13 suppl.): 1325.

184 Goel VK, Deng W, Zhai D et al. Abstract 1444: TPX-0022, a potent MET/SRC/CSF1R inhibitor that modulates the tumor immune microenvironment in preclinical models. Cancer Res 2021; 81 (13 suppl.): 1444.

185 Hong DS, Sen S, Park H et al. A phase I, open-label, multicenter, first-in-human study of the safety, tolerability, pharmacokinetics, and antitumor activity of TPX-0022, a novel MET/CSF1R/SRC inhibitor, in patients with advanced solid tumors harboring genetic alterations in MET. J Clin Oncol 2020; 38 (15 suppl.): TPS3663.

186 Strickler JH, Weekes CD, Nemunaitis J et al. First-in-human phase I, dose-escalation and -expansion study of telisotuzumab vedotin, an antibody-drug conjugate targeting c-Met, in patients with advanced solid tumors. J Clin Oncol 2018; 36 (33): 3298–3306.

187 Strickler JH, LoRusso P, Yen C-J et al. Phase 1, open-label, dose-escalation, and expansion study of ABT-700, an anti-C-met antibody, in patients (pts) with advanced solid tumors. J Clin Oncol 2014; 32 (15 suppl.): 2507.

188 Ocampo C, Wu J, Dey J et al. P2.01–19 phase 2 study of telisotuzumab vedotin (Teliso-V) in previously treated c-MET+ non-small cell lung cancer: Trial in progress. J Thorac Oncol 2019; 14 (10).

189 Spira A, Krebs M, Cho BC et al. OA15.03 amivantamab in non-small cell lung cancer (NSCLC) with *MET exon 14* skipping (METex14) mutation: Initial results from CHRYSALIS. J Thorac Oncol 2021; 16 (10 suppl.): S874–S875.

190 Pantsar T. The current understanding of KRAS protein structure and dynamics. Comput Struct Biotechnol J 2020; 18: 189–198.

191 Ahearn IM, Haigis K, Bar-Sagi D et al. Regulating the regulator: Post-translational modification of RAS. Nat Rev Mol Cell Biol 2011; 13 (1): 39–51.

192 Bos JL, Rehmann H, Wittinghofer A. GEFs and GAPs: Critical elements in the control of small G proteins. Cell 2007; 129 (5): 865–877.

193 Stephen AG, Esposito D, Bagni RK et al. Dragging ras back in the ring. Cancer Cell 2014; 25 (3): 272–281.

194 Prior IA, Hood FE, Hartley JL. The frequency of Ras mutations in cancer. Cancer Res 2020; 80 (14): 2969–2974.

195 Hunter JC, Manandhar A, Carrasco MA et al. Biochemical and structural analysis of common cancer-associated KRAS mutations. Mol Cancer Res 2015; 13 (9): 1325–1335.

196 Molina-Arcas M, Samani A, Downward J. Drugging the undruggable: Advances on RAS targeting in cancer. Genes 2021; 12 (6): 899.

197 Moore AR, Rosenberg SC, McCormick F et al. RAS-targeted therapies: Is the undruggable drugged? Nat Rev Drug Discov 2020; 19 (8): 533–552.

198 Spencer-Smith R, O'Bryan JP. Direct inhibition of RAS: Quest for the Holy Grail? Semin Cancer Biol 2019; 54: 138–148.

199 Blumenschein GR, Smit EF, Planchard D et al. A randomized phase II study of the MEK1/MEK2 inhibitor trametinib (GSK1120212) compared with docetaxel in KRAS-mutant advanced non-small-cell lung cancer (NSCLC)†. Ann Oncol 2015; 26 (5): 894–901.

200 Ostrem JM, Peters U, Sos ML et al. K-RAS(G12C) inhibitors allosterically control GTP affinity and effector interactions. Nature 2013; 503 (7477): 548–551.

201 Lanman BA, Allen JR, Allen JG et al. Discovery of a covalent inhibitor of KRASG12C (AMG 510) for the treatment of solid tumors. J Med Chem 2020; 63 (1): 52–65.

202 Canon J, Rex K, Saiki AY et al. The clinical KRAS(G12C) inhibitor AMG 510 drives anti-tumour immunity. Nature 2019; 575 (7781): 217–223.

203 Hong DS, Fakih MG, Strickler JH et al. KRASG12C inhibition with sotorasib in advanced solid tumors. N Engl J Med 2020; 383 (13): 1207–1217.

204 Skoulidis F, Li BT, Govindan R et al. Overall survival and exploratory subgroup analyses from the phase 2 CodeBreaK 100 trial evaluating

sotorasib in pretreated KRAS p.G12C mutated non-small cell lung cancer. J Clin Oncol 2021; 39 (15 suppl.): 9003.

205 Skoulidis F, Li BT, Dy GK et al. Sotorasib for lung cancers with KRAS p.G12C mutation. N Engl J Med 2021; 384 (25): 2371–2381.

206 Fell JB, Fischer JP, Baer BR et al. Identification of the clinical development candidate MRTX849, a covalent KRASG12C inhibitor for the treatment of cancer. J Med Chem 2020; 63 (13): 6679–6693.

207 Ou SI, Janne PA, Leal TA et al. First-in-human phase I/IB dose-finding study of adagrasib (MRTX849) in patients with advanced KRAS(G12C) solid tumors (KRYSTAL-1). J Clin Oncol 2022; 40 (23): JCO2102752.

208 Koga T, Suda K, Fujino T et al. KRAS secondary mutations that confer acquired resistance to KRAS G12C inhibitors, sotorasib and adagrasib, and overcoming strategies: Insights from in vitro experiments. J Thorac Oncol 2021; 16 (8): 1321–1332.

209 Tanaka N, Lin JJ, Li C et al. Clinical acquired resistance to KRASG12C inhibition through a novel KRAS switch-II pocket mutation and polyclonal alterations converging on RAS-MAPK reactivation. Cancer Discov 2021; 11 (8): 1913–1922.

210 Awad MM, Liu S, Rybkin II et al. Acquired resistance to KRASG12C inhibition in cancer. N Engl J Med 2021; 384 (25): 2382–2393.

211 Jeanson A, Tomasini P, Souquet-Bressand M et al. Efficacy of immune checkpoint inhibitors in KRAS-mutant non-small cell lung cancer (NSCLC). J Thorac Oncol 2019; 14 (6): 1095–1101.

212 Xie M, Xu X, Fan Y. KRAS-mutant non-small cell lung cancer: An emerging promisingly treatable subgroup. Front Oncol 2021; 11: 672612.

213 Gadgeel S, Rodriguez-Abreu D, Felip E et al. KRAS mutational status and efficacy in KEYNOTE-189: Pembrolizumab (pembro) plus chemotherapy (chemo) vs placebo plus chemo as first-line therapy for metastatic non-squamous NSCLC. Ann Oncol 2019; 30: xi64–xi65.

214 Peng S-B, Si C, Zhang Y et al. Abstract 1259: Preclinical characterization of LY3537982, a novel, highly selective and potent KRAS-G12C inhibitor. Cancer Res 2021; 81 (13 suppl.): 1259.

215 Savarese F, Gollner A, Rudolph D et al. Abstract 1271: In vitro and in vivo characterization of BI 1823911 – A novel KRASG12C selective small molecule inhibitor. Cancer Res 2021; 81 (13 suppl.): 1271.

216 Nichols RJ, Cregg J, Schulze CJ et al. Abstract 1261: A next generation tri-complex KRASG12C(ON) inhibitor directly targets the active, GTP-bound state of mutant RAS and may overcome resistance to KRASG12C(OFF) inhibition. Cancer Res 2021; 81 (13 suppl.): 1261.

217 Mainardi S, Mulero-Sánchez A, Prahallad A et al. SHP2 is required for growth of KRAS-mutant non-small-cell lung cancer in vivo. Nat Med 2018; 24 (7): 961–967.

218 Hallin J, Engstrom LD, Hargis L et al. The KRASG12C inhibitor MRTX849 provides insight toward therapeutic susceptibility of KRAS-mutant cancers in mouse models and patients. Cancer Discov 2020; 10 (1): 54–71.

219 Yaeger R, Corcoran RB. Targeting alterations in the RAF-MEK pathway. Cancer Discov 2019; 9 (3): 329–341.

220 Imielinski M, Berger AH, Hammerman PS et al. Mapping the hallmarks of lung adenocarcinoma with massively parallel sequencing. Cell 2012; 150 (6): 1107–1120.

221 Menzies AM, Yeh I, Botton T et al. Clinical activity of the MEK inhibitor trametinib in metastatic melanoma containing BRAF kinase fusion. Pigment Cell Melanoma Res 2015; 28 (5): 607–610.

222 Roskoski R, Jr. RAF protein-serine/threonine kinases: Structure and regulation. Biochem Biophys Res Commun 2010; 399 (3): 313–317.

223 Pratilas CA, Taylor BS, Ye Q et al. (V600E)BRAF is associated with disabled feedback inhibition of RAF-MEK signaling and elevated transcriptional output of the pathway. Proc Natl Acad Sci USA 2009; 106 (11): 4519–4524.

224 Weiss RH, Maga EA, Ramirez A. MEK inhibition augments Raf activity, but has variable effects on mitogenesis, in vascular smooth muscle cells. Am J Physiol 1998; 274 (6): C1521–C1529.

225 Lake D, Correa SA, Muller J. Negative feedback regulation of the ERK1/2 MAPK pathway. Cell Mol Life Sci 2016; 73 (23): 4397–4413.

226 Ho CC, Liao WY, Lin CA et al. Acquired *BRAF* V600E mutation as resistant mechanism after treatment with osimertinib. J Thorac Oncol 2017; 12 (3): 567–572.

227 Lee C, Rhee I. Important roles of protein tyrosine phosphatase PTPN12 in tumor progression. Pharmacol Res 2019; 144: 73–78.

228 Smiech M, Leszczynski P, Kono H et al. Emerging *BRAF* mutations in cancer progression and their possible effects on transcriptional networks. Genes (Basel) 2020; 11 (11).

229 Wan PTC, Garnett MJ, Roe SM et al. Mechanism of activation of the RAF-ERK signaling pathway by oncogenic mutations of B-RAF. Cell 2004; 116 (6): 855–867.

230 Kobayashi M, Sonobe M, Takahashi T et al. Clinical significance of BRAF gene mutations in patients with non-small cell lung cancer. Anticancer Res 2011; 31 (12): 4619–4623.

231 Davies H, Bignell GR, Cox C et al. Mutations of the *BRAF* gene in human cancer. Nature 2002; 417 (6892): 949–954.

232 Brose MS, Volpe P, Feldman M et al. BRAF and RAS mutations in human lung cancer and melanoma. Cancer Res 2002; 62 (23): 6997–7000.

233 Bracht JWP, Karachaliou N, Bivona T et al. BRAF mutations classes I, II, and III in NSCLC patients included in the SLLIP trial: The need for a new pre-clinical treatment rationale. Cancers (Basel) 2019; 11 (9).

234 Roviello G, D'Angelo A, Sirico M et al. Advances in anti-BRAF therapies for lung cancer. Invest New Drugs 2021; 39 (3): 879–890.

235 Pratilas CA, Hanrahan AJ, Halilovic E et al. Genetic predictors of MEK dependence in non-small cell lung cancer. Cancer Res 2008; 68 (22): 9375–9383.

236 Paik PK, Arcila ME, Fara M et al. Clinical characteristics of patients with lung adenocarcinomas harboring BRAF mutations. J Clin Oncol 2011; 29 (15): 2046–2051.

237 Tan I, Stinchcombe TE, Ready NE et al. Therapeutic outcomes in non-small cell lung cancer with BRAF mutations: A single institution, retrospective cohort study. Transl Lung Cancer Res 2019; 8 (3): 258–267.

238 Sheikine Y, Pavlick D, Klempner SJ et al. BRAF in lung cancers: Analysis of patient cases reveals recurrent *BRAF* mutations, fusions, kinase duplications, and concurrent alterations. JCO Precis Oncol 2018; 2.

239 Vojnic M, Kubota D, Kurzatkowski C et al. Acquired BRAF rearrangements induce secondary resistance to EGFR therapy in EGFR-mutated lung cancers. J Thorac Oncol 2019; 14 (5): 802–815.

240 Frisone D, Friedlaender A, Malapelle U et al. A BRAF new world. Crit Rev Oncol Hematol 2020; 152: 103008.

241 Dagogo-Jack I, Martinez P, Yeap BY et al. Impact of BRAF mutation class on disease characteristics and clinical outcomes in BRAF-mutant lung cancer. Clin Cancer Res 2019; 25 (1): 158–165.

242 Yousem SA, Nikiforova M, Nikiforov Y. The histopathology of *BRAF*-V600E-mutated lung adenocarcinoma. Am J Surg Pathol 2008; 32 (9): 1317–1321.

243 Marchetti A, Felicioni L, Malatesta S et al. Clinical features and outcome of patients with non-small-cell lung cancer harboring BRAF mutations. J Clin Oncol 2011; 29 (26): 3574–3579.

244 Cardarella S, Ogino A, Nishino M et al. Clinical, pathologic, and biologic features associated with BRAF mutations in non-small cell lung cancer. Clin Cancer Res 2013; 19 (16): 4532–4540.

245 Planchard D, Besse B, Groen HJM et al. Dabrafenib plus trametinib in patients with previously treated BRAFV600E-mutant metastatic non-small

cell lung cancer: An open-label, multicentre phase 2 trial. Lancet Oncol 2016; 17 (7): 984–993.

246 Jones JC, Renfro LA, Al-Shamsi HO et al. (Non-V600) BRAF mutations define a clinically distinct molecular subtype of metastatic colorectal cancer. J Clin Oncol 2017; 35 (23): 2624–2630.

247 Reddy VP, Gay LM, Elvin JA et al. BRAF fusions in clinically advanced non-small cell lung cancer: An emerging target for anti-BRAF therapies. J Clin Oncol 2017; 35 (15 suppl.): 9072.

248 Zhao J, Guo R, Ai X et al. BRAF fusion in lung cancer. J Clin Oncol 2020; 38 (15 suppl.): e21598.

249 Wang CY, Hsia JY, Li CH et al. Lung adenocarcinoma With primary LIMD1-BRAF fusion treated with MEK inhibitor: A case report. Clin Lung Cancer 2021; 22 (6): e878–e880.

250 Robert C, Karaszewska B, Schachter J et al. Improved overall survival in melanoma with combined dabrafenib and trametinib. N Engl J Med 2015; 372 (1): 30–39.

251 Grob JJ, Amonkar MM, Karaszewska B et al. Comparison of dabrafenib and trametinib combination therapy with vemurafenib monotherapy on health-related quality of life in patients with unresectable or metastatic cutaneous BRAF Val600-mutation-positive melanoma (COMBI-v): Results of a phase 3, open-label, randomised trial. Lancet Oncol 2015; 16 (13): 1389–1398.

252 Poulikakos PI, Zhang C, Bollag G et al. RAF inhibitors transactivate RAF dimers and ERK signalling in cells with wild-type BRAF. Nature 2010; 464 (7287): 427–430.

253 Sturm OE, Orton R, Grindlay J et al. The mammalian MAPK/ERK pathway exhibits properties of a negative feedback amplifier. Sci Signal 2010; 3 (153): ra90.

254 Hatzivassiliou G, Song K, Yen I et al. RAF inhibitors prime wild-type RAF to activate the MAPK pathway and enhance growth. Nature 2010; 464 (7287): 431–435.

255 Heidorn SJ, Milagre C, Whittaker S et al. Kinase-dead BRAF and oncogenic RAS cooperate to drive tumor progression through CRAF. Cell 2010; 140 (2): 209–221.

256 Flaherty KT, Puzanov I, Kim KB et al. Inhibition of mutated, activated BRAF in metastatic melanoma. N Engl J Med 2010; 363 (9): 809–819.

257 Su F, Viros A, Milagre C et al. RAS mutations in cutaneous squamous-cell carcinomas in patients treated with BRAF inhibitors. N Engl J Med 2012; 366 (3): 207–215.

258 Planchard D, Smit EF, Groen HJM et al. Dabrafenib plus trametinib in patients with previously untreated BRAFV600E-mutant metastatic non-small-cell lung cancer: An open-label, phase 2 trial. Lancet Oncol 2017; 18 (10): 1307–1316.

259 Planchard D, Besse B, Kim TM et al. Updated survival of patients (pts) with previously treated BRAF V600E-mutant advanced non-small cell lung cancer (NSCLC) who received dabrafenib (D) or D + trametinib (T) in the phase II BRF113928 study. J Clin Oncol 2017; 35 (15 suppl.): 9075.

260 Planchard D, Besse B, Groen HJM et al. Phase 2 study of dabrafenib plus trametinib in patients with *BRAF* V600E-mutant metastatic NSCLC: Updated 5-year survival rates and genomic analysis. J Thorac Oncol 2022; 17 (1): 103–115.

261 Odogwu L, Mathieu L, Blumenthal G et al. FDA approval summary: Dabrafenib and trametinib for the treatment of metastatic non-small cell lung cancers harboring *BRAF* V600E mutations. Oncologist 2018; 23 (6): 740–745.

262 Larkin J, Ascierto PA, Dreno B et al. Combined vemurafenib and cobimetinib in *BRAF*-mutated melanoma. N Engl J Med 2014; 371 (20): 1867–1876.

263 Subbiah V, Gervais R, Riely G et al. Efficacy of vemurafenib in patients with non-small-cell lung cancer with *BRAF* V600 mutation: An open-label, single-arm cohort of the histology-independent VE-BASKET study. JCO Precis Oncol 2019; 3.

264 Mazieres J, Cropet C, Montane L et al. Vemurafenib in non-small-cell lung cancer patients with *BRAF*(V600) and *BRAF*(nonV600) mutations. Ann Oncol 2020; 31 (2): 289–294.

265 Gautschi O, Milia J, Cabarrou B et al. Targeted therapy for patients with BRAF-mutant lung cancer: Results from the European EURAF cohort. J Thorac Oncol 2015; 10 (10): 1451–1457.

266 Nebhan CA, Johnson DB, Sullivan RJ et al. Efficacy and safety of trametinib in non-*V600* BRAF mutant melanoma: A phase II study. Oncologist 2021; 26 (9): 731–e1498.

267 Johnson DB, Zhao F, Noel M et al. Trametinib activity in patients with solid tumors and lymphomas harboring *BRAF* non-V600 mutations or fusions: Results from NCI-MATCH (EAY131). Clin Cancer Res 2020; 26 (8): 1812–1819.

268 Dankner M, Lajoie M, Moldoveanu D et al. Dual MAPK inhibition is an effective therapeutic strategy for a subset of class II *BRAF* mutant melanomas. Clin Cancer Res 2018; 24 (24): 6483–6494.

269 Noeparast A, Teugels E, Giron P et al. Non-V600 *BRAF* mutations recurrently found in lung cancer predict sensitivity to the combination of trametinib and dabrafenib. Oncotarget 2017; 8 (36): 60094–60108.

270 Alvarez JGB, Otterson GA. Agents to treat BRAF-mutant lung cancer. Drugs Context 2019; 8: 212566.

271 Reyes R, Mayo-de-Las-Casas C, Teixido C et al. Clinical benefit from BRAF/MEK inhibition in a double non-V600E *BRAF* mutant lung adenocarcinoma: A case report. Clin Lung Cancer 2019; 20 (3): e219–e223.

272 Turshudzhyan A, Vredenburgh J. A rare p.T599dup *BRAF* mutant NSCLC in a non-smoker. Curr Oncol 2020; 28 (1): 196–202.

273 Negrao MV, Raymond VM, Lanman RB et al. Molecular landscape of *BRAF*-mutant NSCLC reveals an association between clonality and driver mutations and identifies targetable non-V600 driver mutations. J Thorac Oncol 2020; 15 (10): 1611–1623.

274 Dudnik E, Peled N, Nechushtan H et al. BRAF mutant lung cancer: Programmed death ligand 1 expression, tumor mutational burden, microsatellite instability status, and response to immune check-point inhibitors. J Thorac Oncol 2018; 13 (8): 1128–1137.

275 Guisier F, Dubos-Arvis C, Vinas F et al. Efficacy and safety of anti-PD-1 immunotherapy in patients with advanced NSCLC with BRAF, HER2, or MET mutations or RET translocation: GFPC 01–2018. J Thorac Oncol 2020; 15 (4): 628–636.

276 Mazieres J, Drilon AE, Mhanna L et al. Efficacy of immune-checkpoint inhibitors (ICI) in non-small cell lung cancer (NSCLC) patients harboring activating molecular alterations (ImmunoTarget). J Clin Oncol 2018; 36 (15 suppl.): 9010.

277 Sullivan RJ, Hollebecque A, Flaherty KT et al. A phase I study of LY3009120, a pan-RAF inhibitor, in patients with advanced or metastatic cancer. Mol Cancer Ther 2020; 19 (2): 460–467.

278 Paraiso KH, Xiang Y, Rebecca VW et al. PTEN loss confers BRAF inhibitor resistance to melanoma cells through the suppression of BIM expression. Cancer Res 2011; 71 (7): 2750–2760.

279 Manzano JL, Layos L, Buges C et al. Resistant mechanisms to BRAF inhibitors in melanoma. Ann Transl Med 2016; 4 (12): 237.

280 Gibney GT, Smalley KS. An unholy alliance: Cooperation between BRAF and NF1 in melanoma development and BRAF inhibitor resistance. Cancer Discov 2013; 3 (3): 260–263.

281 Carlino MS, Fung C, Shahheydari H et al. Preexisting MEK1P124 mutations diminish response to BRAF inhibitors in metastatic melanoma patients. Clin Cancer Res 2015; 21 (1): 98–105.

282 Nassar KW, Hintzsche JD, Bagby SM et al. Targeting CDK4/6 represents a therapeutic vulnerability in acquired BRAF/MEK inhibitor-resistant melanoma. Mol Cancer Ther 2021; 20 (10): 2049–2060.

283 Yao Z, Torres NM, Tao A et al. BRAF mutants evade ERK-dependent feedback by different mechanisms that determine their sensitivity to pharmacologic inhibition. Cancer Cell 2015; 28 (3): 370–383.

284 Corcoran RB, Ebi H, Turke AB et al. EGFR-mediated re-activation of MAPK signaling contributes to insensitivity of BRAF mutant colorectal cancers to RAF inhibition with vemurafenib. Cancer Discov 2012; 2 (3): 227–235.

285 Prahallad A, Sun C, Huang S et al. Unresponsiveness of colon cancer to BRAF(V600E) inhibition through feedback activation of EGFR. Nature 2012; 483 (7387): 100–103.

286 Abravanel DL, Nishino M, Sholl LM et al. An acquired NRAS Q61K mutation in *BRAF* V600E-mutant lung adenocarcinoma resistant to dabrafenib plus trametinib. J Thorac Oncol 2018; 13 (8): e131–e133.

287 Facchinetti F, Lacroix L, Mezquita L et al. Molecular mechanisms of resistance to BRAF and MEK inhibitors in BRAF(V600E) non-small cell lung cancer. Eur J Cancer 2020; 132: 211–223.

288 Niemantsverdriet M, Schuuring E, Elst AT et al. KRAS mutation as a resistance mechanism to BRAF/MEK inhibition in NSCLC. J Thorac Oncol 2018; 13 (12): e249–e251.

289 Rudin CM, Hong K, Streit M. Molecular characterization of acquired resistance to the BRAF inhibitor dabrafenib in a patient with BRAF-mutant non-small-cell lung cancer. J Thorac Oncol 2013; 8 (5): e41–42.

290 Schrock AB, Zhu VW, Hsieh WS et al. Receptor tyrosine kinase fusions and BRAF kinase fusions are rare but actionable resistance mechanisms to EGFR tyrosine kinase inhibitors. J Thorac Oncol 2018; 13 (9): 1312–1323.

291 Huang Y, Gan J, Guo K et al. Acquired BRAF V600E mutation mediated resistance to osimertinib and responded to osimertinib, dabrafenib, and trametinib combination therapy. J Thorac Oncol 2019; 14 (10): e236–e237.

292 Meng P, Koopman B, Kok K et al. Combined osimertinib, dabrafenib and trametinib treatment for advanced non-small-cell lung cancer patients with an osimertinib-induced BRAF V600E mutation. Lung Cancer 2020; 146: 358–361.

293 Solassol J, Vendrell JA, Senal R et al. Challenging BRAF/EGFR co-inhibition in NSCLC using sequential liquid biopsies. Lung Cancer 2019; 133: 45–47.

294 Zhou F, Zhao W, Chen X et al. Response to the combination of dabrafenib, trametinib and osimertinib in a patient with EGFR-mutant NSCLC harboring an acquired BRAF(V600E) mutation. Lung Cancer 2020; 139: 219–220.

295 Dagogo-Jack I, Piotrowska Z, Cobb R et al. Response to the combination of osimertinib and trametinib in a patient with EGFR-mutant NSCLC harboring an acquired BRAF fusion. J Thorac Oncol 2019; 14 (10): e226–e228.

296 Ross JS, Wang K, Chmielecki J et al. The distribution of *BRAF* gene fusions in solid tumors and response to targeted therapy. Int J Cancer 2016; 138 (4): 881–890.

297 Okimoto RA, Lin L, Olivas V et al. Preclinical efficacy of a RAF inhibitor that evades paradoxical MAPK pathway activation in protein kinase BRAF-mutant lung cancer. Proc Natl Acad Sci USA 2016; 113 (47): 13456–13461.

298 Yao Z, Gao Y, Su W et al. RAF inhibitor PLX8394 selectively disrupts BRAF dimers and RAS-independent BRAF-mutant-driven signaling. Nat Med 2019; 25 (2): 284–291.

299 Koumaki K, Kontogianni G, Kosmidou V et al. BRAF paradox breakers PLX8394, PLX7904 are more effective against BRAFV600Epsilon CRC cells compared with the BRAF inhibitor PLX4720 and shown by detailed pathway analysis. Biochim Biophys Acta Mol Basis Dis 2021; 1867 (4): 166061.

300 Janku F, Sherman EJ, Parikh AR et al. Interim results from a phase 1/2 precision medicine study of PLX8394: A next generation BRAF inhibitor. Eur J Cancer 2020; 138: S2–S3.

301 Kim TW, Lee J, Shin SJ et al. Belvarafenib, a novel pan-RAF inhibitor, in solid tumor patients harboring BRAF, KRAS, or NRAS mutations: Phase I study. J Clin Oncol 2019; 37 (15 suppl.): 3000.

302 Varga A, Soria JC, Hollebecque A et al. A first-in-human phase I study to evaluate the ERK1/2 inhibitor GDC-0994 in patients with advanced solid tumors. Clin Cancer Res 2020; 26 (6): 1229–1236.

303 Moschos SJ, Sullivan RJ, Hwu WJ et al. Development of MK-8353, an orally administered ERK1/2 inhibitor, in patients with advanced solid tumors. JCI Insight 2018; 3 (4).

304 Sullivan RJ, Infante JR, Janku F et al. First-in-class ERK1/2 inhibitor ulixertinib (BVD-523) in patients with MAPK mutant advanced solid tumors: Results of a phase I dose-escalation and expansion study. Cancer Discov 2018; 8 (2): 184–195.

305 Desai J, Gan H, Barrow C et al. Phase I, open-label, dose-escalation/ dose-expansion study of lifirafenib (BGB-283), an RAF family kinase

inhibitor, in patients with solid tumors. J Clin Oncol 2020; 38 (19): 2140–2150.

306 Pulciani S, Santos E, Lauver AV et al. Oncogenes in solid human tumours. Nature 1982; 300 (5892): 539–542.

307 Martin-Zanca D, Hughes SH, Barbacid M. A human oncogene formed by the fusion of truncated tropomyosin and protein tyrosine kinase sequences. Nature 1986; 319 (6056): 743–748.

308 Valent A, Danglot G, Bernheim A. Mapping of the tyrosine kinase receptors trkA (NTRK1), trkB (NTRK2) and trkC(NTRK3) to human chromosomes 1q22, 9q22 and 15q25 by fluorescence in situ hybridization. Eur J Hum Genet 1997; 5 (2): 102–104.

309 Chao MV. Neurotrophins and their receptors: A convergence point for many signalling pathways. Nat Rev Neurosci 2003; 4 (4): 299–309.

310 Stransky N, Cerami E, Schalm S et al. The landscape of kinase fusions in cancer. Nat Commun 2014; 5: 4846.

311 Cocco E, Scaltriti M, Drilon A. NTRK fusion-positive cancers and TRK inhibitor therapy. Nat Rev Clin Oncol 2018; 15 (12): 731–747.

312 Tognon C GM, Kenward E, Kay R, Morrison K, Sorensen PH. The chimeric protein tyrosine kinase ETV6-NTRK3 requires both Ras-Erk1/2 and PI3-kinase-Akt signaling for fibroblast transformation. Cancer Res 2001; 61 (24): 8909–8916.

313 Ozono K, Ohishi Y, Onishi H et al. Brain-derived neurotrophic factor/tropomyosin-related kinase B signaling pathway contributes to the aggressive behavior of lung squamous cell carcinoma. Lab Invest 2017; 97 (11): 1332–1342.

314 Greco A, Miranda C, Pierotti MA. Rearrangements of *NTRK1* gene in papillary thyroid carcinoma. Mol Cell Endocrinol 2010; 321 (1): 44–49.

315 Shah N, Lankerovich M, Lee H et al. Exploration of the gene fusion landscape of glioblastoma using transcriptome sequencing and copy number data. BMC Genomics 2013; 14: 818.

316 Ross JS, Wang K, Gay L et al. New routes to targeted therapy of intrahepatic cholangiocarcinomas revealed by next-generation sequencing. Oncologist 2014; 19 (3): 235–242.

317 Marchio C, Scaltriti M, Ladanyi M et al. ESMO recommendations on the standard methods to detect NTRK fusions in daily practice and clinical research. Ann Oncol 2019; 30 (9): 1417–1427.

318 Vaishnavi A, Capelletti M, Le AT et al. Oncogenic and drug-sensitive NTRK1 rearrangements in lung cancer. Nat Med 2013; 19 (11): 1469–1472.

319 Farago AF, Taylor MS, Doebele RC et al. Clinicopathologic features of non-small-cell lung cancer harboring an NTRK gene fusion. JCO Precis Oncol 2018; 2018.

320 Okamura K, Harada T, Wang S et al. Expression of TrkB and BDNF is associated with poor prognosis in non-small cell lung cancer. Lung Cancer 2012; 78 (1): 100–106.

321 Ekman S. How selecting best therapy for metastatic NTRK fusion-positive non-small cell lung cancer? Transl Lung Cancer Res 2020; 9 (6): 2535–2544.

322 Drilon A, Laetsch TW, Kummar S et al. Efficacy of larotrectinib in TRK fusion-positive cancers in adults and children. N Engl J Med 2018; 378 (8): 731–739.

323 Hong DS, DuBois SG, Kummar S et al. Larotrectinib in patients with TRK fusion-positive solid tumours: a pooled analysis of three phase 1/2 clinical trials. Lancet Oncol 2020; 21 (4): 531–540.

324 Drilon A MGV, Patel J, et al. Efficacy and safety of larotrectinib in patients with tropomyosin receptor kinase (TRK) fusion lung cancer. Ann Oncol 2020; 31 (suppl. 4): S754–S840.

325 Haratake N, Seto T. NTRK fusion-positive non–small-cell lung cancer: The diagnosis and targeted therapy. Clin Lung Cancer 2021; 22 (1): 1–5.

326 Doebele RC, Drilon A, Paz-Ares L et al. Entrectinib in patients with advanced or metastatic NTRK fusion-positive solid tumours: Integrated analysis of three phase 1–2 trials. Lancet Oncol 2020; 21 (2): 271–282.

327 Drilon A, Paz-Ares L, Doebele RC et al. 543P Entrectinib in NTRK fusion-positive NSCLC: Updated integrated analysis of STARTRK-2, STARTRK-1 and ALKA-372–001. Ann Oncol 2020; 31: S474–S475.

328 Russo M, Misale S, Wei G et al. Acquired resistance to the TRK inhibitor entrectinib in colorectal cancer. Cancer Discov 2016; 6 (1): 36–44.

329 Drilon A, Li G, Dogan S et al. What hides behind the MASC: Clinical response and acquired resistance to entrectinib after ETV6-NTRK3 identification in a mammary analogue secretory carcinoma (MASC). Ann Oncol 2016; 27 (5): 920–926.

330 Doebele RC DR, Drilon A, et al. Genomic landscape of entrectinib resistance from ctDNA analysis in STARTRK-2. Ann Oncol 2019;30; 30 (suppl. 5): v865.

331 Fuse MJ, Okada K, Oh-Hara T et al. Mechanisms of resistance to NTRK inhibitors and therapeutic strategies in *NTRK1*-rearranged cancers. Mol Cancer Ther 2017; 16 (10): 2130–2143.

332 Russo A, Cardona AF, Caglevic C et al. Overcoming TKI resistance in fusion-driven NSCLC: New generation inhibitors and rationale for combination strategies. Transl Lung Cancer Res 2020; 9 (6): 2581–2598.

333 Poh A. Combating acquired TRK inhibitor resistance. Cancer Discov 2019; 9 (6): 684–685.

334 Hyman D, Kummar S, Farago A et al. Abstract CT127: Phase I and expanded access experience of LOXO-195 (BAY 2731954), a selective next-generation TRK inhibitor (TRKi). Cancer Res 2019; 79 (13 suppl.): CT127.

335 Drilon A, Ou SI, Cho BC et al. Repotrectinib (TPX-0005) is a next-generation ROS1/TRK/ALK inhibitor that potently inhibits ROS1/TRK/ALK solvent-front mutations. Cancer Discov 2018; 8 (10): 1227–1236.

336 Drilon AZD, Zhai D, Deng W et al. Repotrectinib, a next generation TRK inhibitor, overcomes TRK resistance mutations including solvent front, gatekeeper and compound mutations. Cancer Res 2019; 79 (13 suppl.): 442.

337 Cho BC DR, Lin JJ, et al. Phase 1/2 TRIDENT-1 study of repotrectinib in patients with ROS1+ or NTRK+ advanced solid tumors. *International Association for the Study of Lung Cancer 2020 World Conference on Lung Cancer*. Abstract MA11.07. 2021 (virtual).

338 Zhou C, Zhou H, Yan B. Innovent and AnHeart announce interim data from phase 2 trial (TRUST study) of taletrectinib in ROS1-positive NSCLC at the CSCO 2021 Annual Meeting. Innovent Biologics Inc., Suzhou, September 27, 2021.

339 Wieduwilt MJ, Moasser MM. The epidermal growth factor receptor family: Biology driving targeted therapeutics. Cell Mol Life Sci 2008; 65 (10): 1566–1584.

340 Yarden Y. Biology of HER2 and its importance in breast cancer. Oncology 2001; 61 (suppl. 2): 1–13.

341 Nakamura H, Saji H, Ogata A et al. Correlation between encoded protein overexpression and copy number of the *HER2* gene with survival in non-small cell lung cancer. Intern J Cancer 2003; 103 (1): 61–66.

342 Zhao J, Xia Y. Targeting HER2 alterations in non–small-cell lung cancer: A comprehensive review. JCO Precis Oncol 2020 (4): 411–425.

343 Liu L, Shao X, Gao W et al. The role of human epidermal growth factor receptor 2 as a prognostic factor in lung cancer: A meta-analysis of published data. J Thorac Oncol 2010; 5 (12): 1922–1932.

344 Yoshizawa A, Sumiyoshi S, Sonobe M et al. HER2 status in lung adeno-carcinoma: A comparison of immunohistochemistry, fluorescence in situ hybridization (FISH), dual-ISH, and gene mutations. Lung Cancer 2014; 85 (3): 373–378.

345 Greulich H, Kaplan B, Mertins P et al. Functional analysis of receptor tyrosine kinase mutations in lung cancer identifies oncogenic extracellular

domain mutations of ERBB2. Proc Natl Acad Sci USA 2012; 109 (36): 14476–14481.

346 Patil T, Mushtaq R, Marsh S et al. Clinicopathologic characteristics, treatment outcomes, and acquired resistance patterns of atypical EGFR mutations and HER2 alterations in stage IV non-small-cell lung cancer. Clin Lung Cancer 2020; 21 (3): e191–e204.

347 Arcila ME, Chaft JE, Nafa K et al. Prevalence, clinicopathologic associations, and molecular spectrum of ERBB2 (HER2) tyrosine kinase mutations in lung adenocarcinomas. Clin Cancer Res 2012; 18 (18): 4910–4918.

348 Mazières J, Barlesi F, Filleron T et al. Lung cancer patients with HER2 mutations treated with chemotherapy and HER2-targeted drugs: Results from the European EUHER2 cohort. Ann Oncol 2016; 27 (2): 281–286.

349 De Grève J, Moran T, Graas M-P et al. Phase II study of afatinib, an irreversible ErbB family blocker, in demographically and genotypically defined lung adenocarcinoma. Lung Cancer 2015; 88 (1): 63–69.

350 Dziadziuszko R, Smit EF, Dafni U et al. Afatinib in NSCLC With HER2 mutations: Results of the prospective, open-label phase II NICHE trial of European Thoracic Oncology Platform (ETOP). J Thorac Oncol 2019; 14 (6): 1086–1094.

351 Kris MG, Camidge DR, Giaccone G et al. Targeting HER2 aberrations as actionable drivers in lung cancers: phase II trial of the pan-HER tyrosine kinase inhibitor dacomitinib in patients with HER2-mutant or amplified tumors. Ann Oncol 2015; 26 (7): 1421–1427.

352 Hyman DM, Piha-Paul SA, Won H et al. HER kinase inhibition in patients with HER2- and HER3-mutant cancers. Nature 2018; 554 (7691): 189–194.

353 Gandhi L, Besse B, Mazieres J et al. MA04.02 neratinib ± temsirolimus in HER2-mutant lung cancers: An international, randomized phase II study. J Thorac Oncol 2017; 12 (1 suppl.): S358–S359.

354 Kim TM, Lee K-W, Oh D-Y et al. Phase 1 studies of poziotinib, an irreversible pan-HER tyrosine kinase inhibitor in patients with advanced solid tumors. Cancer Res Treat 2018; 50 (3): 835–842.

355 Elamin YY, Robichaux JP, Carter BW et al. Poziotinib for patients with HER2 exon 20 Mutant non-small-cell lung cancer: Results from a phase II trial. J Clin Oncol 2021: JCO2101113.

356 Socinski MA, Cornelissen R, Garassino MC et al. LBA60 ZENITH20, a multinational, multi-cohort phase II study of poziotinib in NSCLC patients with EGFR or HER2 exon 20 insertion mutations. Ann Oncol 2020; 31: S1188.

357 Riudavets M, Sullivan I, Abdayem P et al. Targeting HER2 in non-small-cell lung cancer (NSCLC): A glimpse of hope? An updated review on therapeutic strategies in NSCLC harbouring HER2 alterations. ESMO Open 2021; 6 (5): 100260.

358 Wang Y, Jiang T, Qin Z et al. HER2 exon 20 insertions in non-small-cell lung cancer are sensitive to the irreversible pan-HER receptor tyrosine kinase inhibitor pyrotinib. Ann Oncol 2019; 30 (3): 447–455.

359 Zhou C, Li X, Wang Q et al. Pyrotinib in HER2-mutant advanced lung adenocarcinoma after platinum-based chemotherapy: A multicenter, open-label, single-arm, phase II study. J Clin Oncol 2020; 38 (24): 2753–2761.

360 Kinoshita I, Goda T, Watanabe K et al. A phase II study of trastuzumab monotherapy in pretreated patients with non-small cell lung cancers (NSCLCs) harboring HER2 alterations: HOT1303-B trial. Ann Oncol 2018; 29: viii540.

361 Gatzemeier U, Groth G, Butts C et al. Randomized phase II trial of gemcitabine-cisplatin with or without trastuzumab in HER2-positive non-small-cell lung cancer. Ann Oncol 2004; 15 (1): 19–27.

362 Hainsworth JD, Meric-Bernstam F, Swanton C et al. Targeted therapy for advanced solid tumors on the basis of molecular profiles: Results from MyPathway, an open-label, phase IIa multiple basket study. J Clin Oncol 2018; 36 (6): 536–542.

363 Hotta K, Aoe K, Kozuki T et al. A phase II study of trastuzumab emtansine in HER2-positive non-small cell lung cancer. J Thorac Oncol 2018; 13 (2): 273–279.

364 Li BT, Shen R, Buonocore D et al. Ado-trastuzumab emtansine for patients with HER2-mutant lung cancers: Results from a phase II basket trial. J Clin Oncol 2018; 36 (24): 2532–2537.

365 Ogitani Y, Aida T, Hagihara K et al. DS-8201a, a novel HER2-targeting ADC with a novel DNA topoisomerase I inhibitor, demonstrates a promising antitumor efficacy with differentiation from T-DM1. Clin Cancer Res 2016; 22 (20): 5097–5108.

366 Tsurutani J, Iwata H, Krop I et al. Targeting HER2 with trastuzumab deruxtecan: A dose-expansion, phase I study in multiple advanced solid tumors. Cancer Discov 2020; 10 (5): 688–701.

367 Li BT, Smit EF, Goto Y et al. Trastuzumab deruxtecan in HER2-mutant non-small-cell lung cancer. N Engl J Med 2021; 386 (3): 241–251.

368 Cheng H, Liu P, Ohlson C et al. PIK3CA(H1047R)- and Her2-initiated mammary tumors escape PI3K dependency by compensatory activation of MEK-ERK signaling. Oncogene 2016; 35 (23): 2961–2970.

369 Zeng J, Ma W, Young RB et al. Targeting HER2 genomic alterations in non-small cell lung cancer. J Nat Cancer Center 2021; 1 (2): 58–73.

370 Song Z, Lv D, Chen S et al. Efficacy and resistance of afatinib in Chinese non-small cell lung cancer patients with HER2 alterations: A multicenter retrospective study. Front Oncol 2021; 11: 657283.

371 Li BT, Michelini F, Misale S et al. HER2-mediated internalization of cytotoxic agents in ERBB2 amplified or mutant lung cancers. Cancer Discov 2020; 10 (5): 674–687.

372 Robichaux JP, Elamin YY, Tan Z et al. Mechanisms and clinical activity of an EGFR and HER2 exon 20-selective kinase inhibitor in non-small cell lung cancer. Nat Med 2018; 24 (5): 638–646.

373 D'Amico L, Menzel U, Prummer M et al. A novel anti-HER2 anthracycline-based antibody-drug conjugate induces adaptive anti-tumor immunity and potentiates PD-1 blockade in breast cancer. J Immunother Cancer 2019; 7 (1): 16.

374 Lindeman NI, Cagle PT, Aisner DL et al. Updated Molecular testing guideline for the selection of lung cancer patients for treatment with targeted tyrosine kinase inhibitors: Guideline from the College of American Pathologists, the International Association for the Study of Lung Cancer, and the Association for Molecular Pathology. Arch Pathol Lab Med 2018; 142 (3): 321–346.

375 Sholl LM, Weremowicz S, Gray SW et al. Combined use of ALK immunohistochemistry and FISH for optimal detection of *ALK*-rearranged lung adenocarcinomas. J Thorac Oncol 2013; 8 (3): 322–328.

376 Go H, Jung YJ, Kang HW et al. Diagnostic method for the detection of KIF5B-RET transformation in lung adenocarcinoma. Lung Cancer 2013; 82 (1): 44–50.

377 Yoshida A, Tsuta K, Wakai S et al. Immunohistochemical detection of ROS1 is useful for identifying ROS1 rearrangements in lung cancers. Mod Pathol 2014; 27 (5): 711–720.

378 Boyle TA, Masago K, Ellison KE et al. ROS1 immunohistochemistry among major genotypes of non-small-cell lung cancer. Clin Lung Cancer 2015; 16 (2): 106–111.

379 Mescam-Mancini L, Lantuejoul S, Moro-Sibilot D et al. On the relevance of a testing algorithm for the detection of *ROS1*-rearranged lung adenocarcinomas. Lung Cancer 2014; 83 (2): 168–173.

380 Chen YF, Hsieh MS, Wu SG et al. Clinical and the prognostic characteristics of lung adenocarcinoma patients with ROS1 fusion in comparison with other driver mutations in East Asian populations. J Thorac Oncol 2014; 9 (8): 1171–1179.

381 Lee SE, Lee B, Hong M et al. Comprehensive analysis of RET and ROS1 rearrangement in lung adenocarcinoma. Mod Pathol 2015; 28 (4): 468–479.

382 Matter MS, Chijioke O, Savic S et al. Narrative review of molecular pathways of kinase fusions and diagnostic approaches for their detection in non-small cell lung carcinomas. Transl Lung Cancer Res 2020; 9 (6): 2645–2655.

383 Kitamura A, Hosoda W, Sasaki E et al. Immunohistochemical detection of EGFR mutation using mutation-specific antibodies in lung cancer. Clin Cancer Res 2010; 16 (13): 3349–3355.

384 Ilie M, Long E, Hofman V et al. Diagnostic value of immunohistochemistry for the detection of the BRAFV600E mutation in primary lung adenocarcinoma Caucasian patients. Ann Oncol 2013; 24 (3): 742–748.

385 Sasaki H, Shimizu S, Tani Y et al. Usefulness of immunohistochemistry for the detection of the BRAF V600E mutation in Japanese lung adenocarcinoma. Lung Cancer 2013; 82 (1): 51–54.

386 Schuler M, Berardi R, Lim WT et al. Molecular correlates of response to capmatinib in advanced non-small-cell lung cancer: clinical and biomarker results from a phase I trial. Ann Oncol 2020; 31 (6): 789–797.

387 Spigel DR, Edelman MJ, O'Byrne K et al. Results From the phase III randomized trial of onartuzumab plus erlotinib versus erlotinib in previously treated stage IIIB or IV non-small-cell lung cancer: METLung. J Clin Oncol 2017; 35 (4): 412–420.

388 Neal JW, Dahlberg SE, Wakelee HA et al. Erlotinib, cabozantinib, or erlotinib plus cabozantinib as second-line or third-line treatment of patients with EGFR wild-type advanced non-small-cell lung cancer (ECOG-ACRIN 1512): A randomised, controlled, open-label, multicentre, phase 2 trial. Lancet Oncol 2016; 17 (12): 1661–1671.

389 Guo R, Berry LD, Aisner DL et al. MET IHC is a poor screen for MET amplification or *MET exon 14* mutations in lung adenocarcinomas: Data from a tri-institutional cohort of the Lung Cancer Mutation Consortium. J Thorac Oncol 2019; 14 (9): 1666–1671.

390 Ricciardi GR, Russo A, Franchina T et al. NSCLC and HER2: Between lights and shadows. J Thorac Oncol 2014; 9 (12): 1750–1762.

391 Yoshizawa A, Sumiyoshi S, Sonobe M et al. HER2 status in lung adenocarcinoma: A comparison of immunohistochemistry, fluorescence in situ hybridization (FISH), dual-ISH, and gene mutations. Lung Cancer 2014; 85 (3): 373–378.

392 Rolfo C, Russo A. HER2 mutations in non-small cell lung cancer: A Herculean effort to hit the target. Cancer Discov 2020; 10 (5): 643–645.

393 Hotta K, Aoe K, Kozuki T et al. A phase II study of trastuzumab emtansine in HER2-positive non-small cell lung cancer. J Thorac Oncol 2018; 13 (2): 273–279.

394 Peters S, Stahel R, Bubendorf L et al. Trastuzumab emtansine (T-DM1) in patients with previously treated HER2-overexpressing metastatic non-small cell lung cancer: Efficacy, safety, and biomarkers. Clin Cancer Res 2019; 25 (1): 64–72.

395 Wang R, Hu H, Pan Y et al. RET fusions define a unique molecular and clinicopathologic subtype of non-small-cell lung cancer. J Clin Oncol 2012; 30 (35): 4352–4359.

396 Rebuzzi SE, Zullo L, Rossi G et al. Novel emerging molecular targets in non-small cell lung cancer. Int J Mol Sci 2021; 22 (5).

397 Hsiao SJ, Zehir A, Sireci AN et al. Detection of tumor NTRK gene fusions to identify patients who may benefit from tyrosine kinase (TRK) inhibitor therapy. J Mol Diagn 2019; 21 (4): 553–571.

398 Vallée A, Herbreteau G, Sagan C et al. 1130P anchored multiplex PCR-based targeted sequencing for the detection of fusion transcripts in FFPE samples of non-small cell lung cancer patients. Ann Oncol 2021; 32.

399 Jennings LJ, Arcila ME, Corless C et al. Guidelines for validation of next-generation sequencing-based oncology panels: A joint consensus recommendation of the Association for Molecular Pathology and College of American Pathologists. J Mol Diagn 2017; 19 (3): 341–365.

400 Benayed R, Offin M, Mullaney K et al. High yield of RNA sequencing for targetable kinase fusions in lung adenocarcinomas with no mitogenic driver alteration detected by DNA sequencing and low tumor mutation burden. Clin Cancer Res 2019; 25 (15): 4712–4722.

401 Oxnard GR, Paweletz CP, Kuang Y et al. Noninvasive detection of response and resistance in *EGFR*-mutant lung cancer using quantitative next-generation genotyping of cell-free plasma DNA. Clin Cancer Res 2014; 20 (6): 1698–1705.

402 Garcia J, Wozny AS, Geiguer F et al. Profiling of circulating tumor DNA in plasma of non-small cell lung cancer patients, monitoring of epidermal growth factor receptor p.T790M mutated allelic fraction using beads, emulsion, amplification, and magnetics companion assay and evaluation in future application in mimicking circulating tumor cells. Cancer Med 2019; 8 (8): 3685–3697.

403 Leighl NB, Page RD, Raymond VM et al. Clinical utility of comprehensive cell-free DNA analysis to identify genomic biomarkers in patients with newly diagnosed metastatic non-small cell lung cancer. Clin Cancer Res 2019; 25 (15): 4691–4700.

404 Aggarwal C, Thompson JC, Black TA et al. Clinical implications of plasma-based genotyping with the delivery of personalized therapy in metastatic non-small cell lung cancer. JAMA Oncol 2019; 5 (2): 173–180.

405 Park S, Lee JC, Choi CM. Clinical applications of liquid biopsy in non-small cell lung cancer patients: Current status and recent advances in clinical practice. J Clin Med 2021; 10 (11).

406 Maheswaran S, Sequist LV, Nagrath S et al. Detection of mutations in *EGFR* in circulating lung-cancer cells. N Engl J Med 2008; 359 (4): 366–377.

407 Guibert N, Pradines A, Farella M et al. Monitoring *KRAS* mutations in circulating DNA and tumor cells using digital droplet PCR during treatment of KRAS-mutated lung adenocarcinoma. Lung Cancer 2016; 100: 1–4.

408 Mondaca S, Lebow ES, Namakydoust A et al. Clinical utility of next-generation sequencing-based ctDNA testing for common and novel ALK fusions. Lung Cancer 2021; 159: 66–73.

409 Odegaard JI, Vincent JJ, Mortimer S et al. Validation of a plasma-based comprehensive cancer genotyping assay utilizing orthogonal tissue- and plasma-based methodologies. Clin Cancer Res 2018; 24 (15): 3539–3549.

410 Thompson JC, Yee SS, Troxel AB et al. Detection of therapeutically targetable driver and resistance mutations in lung cancer patients by next-generation sequencing of cell-free circulating tumor DNA. Clin Cancer Res 2016; 22 (23): 5772–5782.

411 Hochmair MJ, Buder A, Schwab S et al. Liquid-biopsy-based identification of EGFR T790M mutation-mediated resistance to afatinib treatment in patients with advanced *EGFR* mutation-positive NSCLC, and subsequent response to osimertinib. Target Oncol 2019; 14 (1): 75–83.

412 Del Re M, Crucitta S, Gianfilippo G et al. Understanding the mechanisms of resistance in *EGFR*-positive NSCLC: From tissue to liquid biopsy to guide treatment strategy. Int J Mol Sci 2019; 20 (16).

413 Iacovino M, Ciaramella V, Paragliola F et al. Use of liquid biopsy in monitoring therapeutic resistance in *EGFR* oncogene addicted NSCLC. Explor Target Anti-tumor Ther 2020; 1 (6): 391–400.

414 Lee M, Patel D, Jofre S et al. Large cell neuroendocrine carcinoma transformation as a mechanism of acquired resistance to osimertinib in non-small cell lung cancer: Case report and literature review. Clin Lung Cancer 2021.

415 Bettegowda C, Sausen M, Leary RJ et al. Detection of circulating tumor DNA in early- and late-stage human malignancies. Sci Transl Med 2014; 6 (224): 224ra224.

416 Douillard JY, Ostoros G, Cobo M et al. Gefitinib treatment in EGFR mutated caucasian NSCLC: Circulating-free tumor DNA as a surrogate for determination of EGFR status. J Thorac Oncol 2014; 9 (9): 1345–1353.

417 Thress KS, Brant R, Carr TH et al. *EGFR* mutation detection in ctDNA from NSCLC patient plasma: A cross-platform comparison of leading technologies to support the clinical development of AZD9291. Lung Cancer 2015; 90 (3): 509–515.

418 Remon J, Caramella C, Jovelet C et al. Osimertinib benefit in *EGFR*-mutant NSCLC patients with T790M-mutation detected by circulating tumour DNA. Ann Oncol 2017; 28 (4): 784–790.

419 Luo J, Shen L, Zheng D. Diagnostic value of circulating free DNA for the detection of *EGFR* mutation status in NSCLC: A systematic review and meta-analysis. Sci Rep 2014; 4: 6269.

420 Guo R, Luo J, Chang J et al. MET-dependent solid tumours – Molecular diagnosis and targeted therapy. Nat Rev Clin Oncol 2020; 17 (9): 569–587.

421 Paweletz CP, Sacher AG, Raymond CK et al. Bias-corrected targeted next-generation sequencing for rapid, multiplexed detection of actionable alterations in cell-free DNA from advanced lung cancer patients. Clin Cancer Res 2016; 22 (4): 915–922.

422 Fleischhacker M, Schmidt B. Circulating nucleic acids (CNAs) and cancer – A survey. Biochim Biophys Acta 2007; 1775 (1): 181–232.

423 Guo N, Lou F, Ma Y et al. Circulating tumor DNA detection in lung cancer patients before and after surgery. Sci Rep 2016; 6: 33519.

424 Chen K, Zhang J, Guan T et al. Comparison of plasma to tissue DNA mutations in surgical patients with non-small cell lung cancer. J Thorac Cardiovasc Surg 2017; 154 (3): 1123–1131 e1122.

Cambridge Elements ≡

Molecular Oncology

Edward P. Gelmann

University of Arizona

Dr. Edward P. Gelmann is John Norton Professor of Prostate Cancer Research at the University of Arizona and the University of Arizona Cancer Center. Dr. Gelmann previously headed Divisions of Hematology/Oncology at both Georgetown University and Columbia University. He has been the recipient of NIH, DOD and NIEHS grants for his research that has spanned cancer basic, clinical, and population sciences. Dr. Gelmann's research currently focuses on the early stages of prostate carcinogenesis and the development of novel therapeutics for prostate cancer. He continues to be involved in clinical care and clinical research of genitourinary malignancies. He has an active clinical practice and directs GU clinical research at the Cancer Center. Dr. Gelmann has published extensively and is senior editor of the book *Molecular Oncology: Causes of Cancer and Targets for Treatment* (Cambridge University Press, 2013).

About the Series

Therapeutics in clinical oncology are based increasingly on molecular drivers and hallmarks of cancers. *Elements in Molecular Oncology* provides a timely overview of topics in oncology for researchers and clinicians. By focusing on cancer sites or pathways, this series presents information on the latest findings on cancer causation and treatment.

Cambridge Elements ≡

Molecular Oncology

Elements in the Series

Personalized Drug Screening for Functional Tumor Profiling
Victoria El-Khoury, Tatiana Michel, Hichul Kim, and Yong-Jun Kwon

Therapeutic Targeting of RAS Mutant Cancers
Edward C. Stites, Kendra Paskvan, and Shumei Kato

Targeting Oncogenic Driver Mutations in Lung Cancer
Matthew Lee, Fawzi Abu Rous, Alain Borczuk, Stephen Liu, Shirish Gadgeel, and Balazs Halmos

A full series listing is available at: www.cambridge.org/EMO

Printed in the United States
by Baker & Taylor Publisher Services

Printed in the United States
by Baker & Taylor Publisher Services